W9-BXZ-305

Essential Psychopharmacology of Depression and Bipolar Disorder

Essential Psychopharmacology of Depression and Bipolar Disorder is an invaluable resource for all clinicians involved in the treatment of depression and bipolar disorder. Stressing the basic neuroscience of mood disorders, Stephen Stahl's fully updated, authoritative, illustrated text shows how the various antidepressants and mood stabilizers work and gives new information on the pharmacokinetics of antidepressants, including the role of the cytochrome P450 enzyme system and neuropeptides, among them substance P. The mechanism of action of newer antidepressants, including the latest SSRIs, are also prominently and authoritatively reviewed.

Dr. Stephen M. Stahl is currently Adjunct Professor of Psychiatry at the University of California at San Diego. He has conducted numerous research projects awarded by the National Institute of Mental Health, by the Veterans Administration, and by the pharmaceutical industry as a faculty member at Stanford University, the University of California at Los Angeles, the University of London's Institute of Psychiatry, and currently at the University of California at San Diego. Author of more than 200 articles and chapters, Dr. Stahl is an internationally recognized clinician, researcher, and teacher in psychiatry with subspecialty expertise in psychopharmacology. C.M.E. self-assessment tests are also included.

Reviews of *Essential Psychopharmacology First Edition*

"Firmly grounded in contemporary neuroscience . . . the book also provides an excellent and comprehensive account of the pharmacology of drugs currently used to treat psychiatric disorders. The various chapters are heavily illustrated with excellent diagrams, which ensure that the important concepts of drug action can be thoroughly understood."
Psychological Medicine

". . . superb, authoritative exposition of the fundamentals of neuropsychopharmacology and psychoactive drug therapy. With enviable clarity and succinctness, Stahl and the illustrator cover how psychotropic drugs work and how to use them properly. This masterful production will benefit a broad spectrum of readers, from students to knowledgeable and experienced psychopharmacologists."
Psychiatric Times

"Finally, an elegant and beautiful psychopharmacology text written by a basic scientist who is also a clinician."
Journal of Clinical Psychiatry

"This book is essential reading . . . an excellent and comprehensive account of the pharmacology of the drugs currently used to treat psychiatric disorders, including less commonly covered topics such as cognitive disorders and substance abuse . . . I would thoroughly recommend this book to anyone who works with psychotropic drugs—or who has the task of teaching others about them!"
American Journal of Psychiatry

ESSENTIAL PSYCHOPHARMACOLOGY OF DEPRESSION AND BIPOLAR DISORDER

STEPHEN M. STAHL, M.D., Ph.D.

Director
Clinical Neuroscience Research Center
and
Adjunct Professor of Psychiatry
University of California, San Diego

With Illustrations by
Nancy Muntner

Every effort has been made in preparing this book to provide accurate and up-to-date information that is in accord with accepted standards and practice at the time of publication. Nevertheless, the authors, editors, and publisher can make no warranties that the information contained herein is totally free from error, not least because clinical standards are constantly changing through research and regulation. The authors, editors, and publisher therefore disclaim all liability for direct or consequential damages resulting from the use of material contained in this book. Readers are strongly advised to pay careful attention to information provided by the manufacturer of any drugs that they plan to use.

PUBLISHED BY THE PRESS SYNDICATE OF THE UNIVERSITY OF CAMBRIDGE
The Pitt Building, Trumpington Street, Cambridge CB2 1RP, United Kingdom

CAMBRIDGE UNIVERSITY PRESS
The Edinburgh Building, Cambridge CB2 2RU, United Kingdom
40 West 20th Street, New York, NY 10011-4211, USA
10 Stamford Road, Oakleigh, VIC 3166, Australia
Ruiz de Alarcón 13, 28014 Madrid, Spain
Dock House, The Waterfront, Cape Town 8001, South Africa

http://www.cambridge.org

© Cambridge University Press holds the copyright on the understanding that it shall not at any time assign copyright to anyone else without the written permission of the author, Stephen M. Stahl.

This book is in copyright. Subject to statutory exception and to the provisions of relevant collective licensing agreements, no reproduction of any part may take place without the written permission of Cambridge University Press.

First published 2000
Reprinted 2000, 2001

Printed in the United States of America

Typeset in Garamond

A catalog record for this book is available from the British Library

Library of Congress Cataloging-in-Publication Data is available

Stahl, S. M.
    Essential psychopharmacology of depression and bipolar disorder / Stephen M. Stahl; with illustrations by Nancy Muntner.
       p. ; cm.
    "This booklet is a set of three chapters from the second edition of Essential psychopharmacology" —Pref.
    Includes bibliographical references and index.
    ISBN 0-521-78645-2 (pbk.)
    1. Depression, Mental—Chemotherapy. 2. Manic-depressive illness—Chemotherapy.
    3. Psychopharmacology. I. Stahl, S. M. Essential psychopharmacology. II. Title.
    [DNLM: 1. Depressive Disorder—drug therapy. 2. Antidepressive Agents—therapeutic use.
    3. Bipolar Disorder—drug therapy. 4. Neurotransmitter Uptake Inhibitors—therapeutic use.
WM 207 S781e 2000]
RC537.S735 2000
616.85′27061—dc21
                                                     99-056720

ISBN 0 521 78645 2 Paperback

In memory of Daniel X. Freedman—mentor, colleague, and scientific father.

To Cindy, my wife, best friend, and tireless supporter.

To Jennifer and Victoria, my daughters, for their patience and understanding of the demands of authorship.

CONTENTS

PREFACE

This book is a set of the three chapters from the second edition of *Essential Psychopharmacology* that deal exclusively with depression, bipolar disorders, and their treatment with modern psychopharmacological agents. The knowledge base of psychopharmacology for depression and bipolar disorders has exploded since the first edition of *Essential Psychopharmacology*, and this second edition attempts to reflect these changes. Some would argue that antidepressants have become the fastest growing therapeutic market, the largest therapeutic market, the most expensive therapeutic market, and the market with the most prescribers anywhere in the world and anywhere in medicine. Since all specialties prescribe these medications, with psychiatrists in fact a minority of prescribers, there is intense interest in this area of therapeutics.

Before discussing what the specific contents of this book have to offer in the area of depression and bipolar disorder, it may be useful to point out that this text presents fundamentals of psychopharmacology in simplified and readily readable form. Thus, this material should prepare the reader to consult more sophisticated textbooks as well as the professional literature. The organization of the information here also applies principles of programmed learning for the reader, namely repetition and interaction, which have been shown to enhance retention.

Therefore, it is suggested that novices first approach this text by going through it from beginning to end by reviewing only the color graphics and the legends for these graphics. Virtually everything covered in the text is also covered in the graphics and icons. Once having gone through all the color graphics in these chapters, it is recommended that the reader then go back to the beginning of the book and read the entire text, reviewing the graphics at the same time. Finally, after the text has been read, the entire book can be rapidly reviewed merely by referring to the various color graphics in the book. This mechanism of using the materials will create a certain amount of programmed learning by incorporating the elements of repetition, as well as interaction with visual learning through graphics. Hopefully, the visual concepts learned via graphics will reinforce the written concepts learned from the text.

For those of you who are already familiar with psychopharmacology, this book should provide easy reading from beginning to end. Going back and forth between the text and the graphics should provide interaction. Following a reading of the complete text, it should be simple to review the entire book by going through the graphics once again.

The text is purposely written at a conceptual rather than a pragmatic level and includes ideas that are simplifications and rules, while sacrificing precision and discussion of exceptions to rules. Thus, this is not a text for the sophisticated subspecialist in psychopharmacology. Another limitation of the book is that it is not extensively referenced to original papers but rather to textbooks and reviews, including several of the author's.

Some of the specific information the reader can expect from this book in the first chapter includes an explanation of mood disorders and theories about their biological basis and then an extensive description of the three monoaminergic neurotransmitter systems: namely, serotonin, norepinephrine/noradrenaline, and dopamine. The neurokinin/tachykinin family, including various experimental antidepressants such as substance P antagonists, is also explained.

The treatment of depression is covered in the second and third chapters. For the treatment of depression, there are at least two dozen agents acting by eight independent psychopharmacological mechanisms of action, explained here with icons and color graphics. For bipolar disorders, there are at least a half dozen mood stabilizers similarly portrayed. In the second chapter, the classical antidepressants are covered, including tricyclic antidepressants and monoamine oxidase inhibitors. Also, the five prominent serotonin selective reuptake inhibitors (SSRIs) are discussed, both as a class and as individual agents (fluoxetine, paroxetine, sertaline, fluvoxamine, and citalopram), since together the SSRIs make up over 75% of prescriptions for antidepressants in many countries. This second chapter also covers agents that act on noradrenergic neurotransmission, including bupropion as well as the newly marketed selective agent reboxetine.

The third chapter covers the remaining antidepressants as well as the mood stabilizers: the antidepressants include dual-acting agents such as venlafaxine and mirtazapine, as well as the serotonin antagonist nefazodone; the mood stabilizers include lithium as well as several anticonvulsants. Finally, an extensive discussion of antidepressant combinations for depression and bipolar disorders completes the third chapter for more advanced readers.

Best wishes for your first step on your journey into this fascinating field of psychopharmacology.

STEPHEN M. STAHL

DEPRESSION AND BIPOLAR DISORDERS

In this chapter, the reader will develop a foundation of knowledge about the mood disorders characterized by depression, mania, or both. Included here are descriptions of the leading hypotheses that attempt to explain the biological basis of mood disorders, especially depression. To understand these hypotheses, this chapter will formulate key pharmacological principles that apply to neurons using specific mono-amine neurotransmitters, namely norepinephrine (NE; also called noradrenaline or NA), dopamine (DA), and serotonin (also called 5-hydroxytryptamine or 5HT). We will also briefly introduce neuropeptides related to substance P. This will set the stage for understanding the pharmacological concepts underlying the use of antide-pressant and mood-stabilizing drugs, which will be reviewed in Chapters 2 and 3.

Clinical descriptions and criteria for diagnosis of disorders of mood will only be mentioned in passing. The reader should consult standard reference sources for this material. Here we will discuss how discoveries of various antidepressants have im-pacted the diagnostic criteria for depression and how they may have modified the natural history and course of this illness. The goal of this chapter is to acquaint the reader with current ideas about the clinical and biological aspects of mood disorders in order to be prepared to understand how the various antidepressants and mood stabilizers work.

Clinical Features of Mood Disorders

Description of Mood Disorders

Problems with mood are often called affective disorders. Depression and mania are often seen as opposite ends of an affective or mood spectrum. Classically, mania and depression are "poles" apart, thus generating the terms *unipolar* depression, in which patients just experience the *down* or depressed pole and *bipolar* disorder, in which patients at different times experience either the *up* (manic) pole or the *down* (de-pressed) pole. In practice, however, depression and mania may occur simultaneously, which is called a "mixed" mood state. Mania may also occur in lesser degrees, known as "hypomania," or may switch so fast between mania and depression that it is called "rapid cycling."

Depression is an emotion that is universally experienced by virtually everyone at some time in life. Distinguishing the "normal" emotion of depression from an illness requiring medical treatment is often problematic for those who are not trained in the mental health sciences. Stigma and misinformation in our culture create the widespread popular misconception that mental illness such as depression is not a disease but a deficiency of character, which can be overcome with effort. For example, a survey in the early 1990s of the general population revealed that 71% thought that mental illness was due to emotional weakness; 65% thought it was caused by bad parenting; 45% thought it was the victim's fault and could be willed away; 43% thought that mental illness was incurable; 35% thought it was the consequence of sinful behavior; and only 10% thought it had a biological basis or involved the brain (Table 1–1).

Stigma and misinformation can also extend into medical practice, where many depressed patients present with medically unexplained symptoms. "Somatization" is the term used for such use of physical symptoms to express emotional distress, which may be a major reason for misdiagnosis of mental illness by medical and psycho-

Table 1–1. *Public perceptions of mental illness*

71%	Due to emotional weakness
65%	Caused by bad parenting
45%	Victim's fault; can will it away
43%	Incurable
35%	Consequence of sinful bahavior
10%	Has a biological basis; involves the brain

logical practitioners. Many depressed patients with somatic complaints are considered to have no real or treatable illness and thus are not treated for a psychiatric disorder once medical illnesses are evaluated and ruled out. In reality, however, most patients with diffuse unexplained somatic symptoms in primary care settings either have a treatable psychiatric illness (e.g., anxiety or depressive disorder) or are responding to stressful life events. Such patients do not generally have a genuine somatization disorder in which "their symptoms are really all in their mind."

Given how frequent and treatable the affective illnesses are, if there are a few most important points to make in this textbook, one of them is the need for the reader to know how to recognize and treat these illnesses.

Diagnostic Criteria

Accepted, standardized diagnostic criteria are used to separate "normal" depression caused by disappointment or "having a bad day" from the disorders of mood. Such criteria also are used to distinguish feeling good from feeling "better then good" and so expansive and irritable that the feelings amount to mania. Diagnostic criteria for mood disorders are in constant evolution, with current nosologies being set by the Diagnostic and Statistical Manual of Mental Disorders, Fourth Edition (DSM-IV) (Tables 1–2 and 1–3) in the United States and the International Classification of Diseases, Tenth Edition (ICD-10) in other countries. The reader is referred to these references for the specifics of currently accepted diagnostic criteria.

For our purposes, it is sufficient to recognize that the affective disorders are actually *syndromes*. That is, they are *clusters of symptoms*, only one symptom of which is an abnormality of mood. Certainly the quality of mood, the degree of mood change from the normal (up—mania, or down—depression), and the duration of the abnormal mood are all key features of an affective disorder. In addition, however, clinicians must assess *vegetative features* such as sleep, appetite, weight, and sex drive; *cognitive features* such as attention span, frustration tolerance, memory, negative distortions; *impulse control* such as suicide and homicide; *behavioral features* such as motivation, pleasure, interests, fatigability; and *physical (or somatic) features* such as headaches, stomach aches, and muscle tension (Table 1–4).

Epidemiology and Natural History

In the 1990s, diagnostic criteria for depression began to be applied increasingly to describing the epidemiology and natural history of mood disorders so that the effects

Table 1–2. *DSM IV diagnostic criteria for a major depressive episode*

A. Five (or more) of the following symptoms have been present during the same 2-week period and represent a change from previous functioning; at least one of the symptoms is either (1) depressed mood or (2) loss of interest or pleasure. *Note*: Do not include symptoms that are clearly due to a general medical condition, or mood-incongruent delusions or hallucinations.
  1. Depressed mood most of the day, nearly every day, as indicated by either subjective report (e.g., feels sad or empty) or observation made by others (e.g., appears tearful). *Note*: In children and adolescents, can be irritable mood.
  2. Markedly diminished interest or pleasure in all, or almost all, activities most of the day, nearly every day (as indicated by either subjective account or observation made by others).
  3. Significant weight loss when not dieting or weight gain (e.g., a change of more than 5% of body weight in a month), or decrease or increase in appetite nearly every day. *Note*: In children, consider failure to make expected weight gains.
  4. Insomnia or hypersomnia nearly every day.
  5. Psychomotor agitation or retardation nearly every day (observable by others, not merely subjective feelings of restlessness or being slowed down).
  6. Fatigue or loss of energy nearly every day.
  7. Feelings of worthlessness or excessive or inappropriate guilt (which may be delusional) nearly every day (not merely self-reproach or guilt about being sick).
  8. Diminished ability to think or concentrate, or indecisiveness, nearly every day (either by subjective account or as observed by others).
  9. Recurrent thoughts of death (not just fear of dying), recurrent suicidal ideation without a specific plan, or a suicide attempt or a specific plan for committing suicide.
B. The symptoms do not meet criteria for a mixed episode.
C. The symptoms cause clinically significant distress or impairment in social, occupational, or other important areas of functioning.
D. The symptoms are not due to the direct physiological effects of a substance (e.g., a drug of abuse, a medication, or other treatment) or a general medical condition (e.g., hyperthyroidism).
E. The symptoms are not better accounted for by bereavement (i.e., after the loss of a loved one); the symptoms persist for longer than 2 months or are characterized by marked functional impairment, morbid preoccupation with worthlessness, suicidal ideation, psychotic symptoms, or psychomotor retardation.

of treatments could be better measured. Key questions are: What is the incidence of major depressive disorder versus bipolar disorder? How many people have the condition at the present time, and how many in their lifetimes? Are individuals with mood disorders being identified and treated, and if so, how? Also: What is the outcome of their treatment? What is the natural history of their mood disorder without treatment and how is this affected by treatment?

Answers to these questions are just beginning to evolve (Tables 1–5 through 1–10). For example, the incidence of depression is about 5% of the population, whereas the incidence of bipolar disorder is about 1%. Thus, up to 15 million individuals are currently suffering from depression and another 2 to 3 million from bipolar disorders in the United States. Unfortunately, only about one-third of individuals with depression are in treatment, not only because of underrecognition by health care providers but also because individuals often conceive of their depression as a type of moral deficiency, which is shameful and should be hidden. Individuals often feel as if they could get better if they just "pulled themselves up by the bootstraps"

Table 1–3. *DSM IV diagnostic criteria for a manic episode*

A. A distinct period of abnormally and persistently elevated, expansive, or irritable mood, lasting at least 1 week (or any duration if hospitalization is necessary).
B. During the period of mood disturbance, three (or more) of the following symptoms have persisted (four if the mood is only irritable) and have been present to a significant degree:
    1. Inflated self-esteem or grandiosity.
    2. Decreased need for sleep (e.g., feels rested after only 3 hours of sleep).
    3. More talkative than usual or pressure to keep talking.
    4. Flight of ideas or subjective experience that thoughts are racing.
    5. Distractibility (i.e., attention too easily drawn to unimportant or irrelevant external stimuli).
    6. Increase in goal-directed activity (either socially, at work or school, or sexually) or psychomotor agitation.
    7. Excessive involvement in pleasurable activities that have a high potential for painful consequences (e.g., engaging in unrestrained buying sprees, sexual indiscretions, or foolish business investments).
C. The symptoms do not meet criteria for a mixed episode.
D. The mood disturbance is sufficiently severe to cause marked impairment in occupational functioning or in usual social activities or relationships with others, or to necessitate hospitalization to prevent harm to self or others, or there are psychotic features.
E. The symptoms are not due to the direct physiological effects of a substance (e.g., a drug of abuse, a medication, or other treatment) or a general medical condition (e.g., hyperthyroidism). *Note*: Manic-like episodes that are clearly caused by somatic antidepressant treatment (e.g., medication, electroconvulsive therapy, light therapy) should not count toward a diagnosis of bipolar I disorder.

Table 1–4. *Depression is a syndrome*

Clusters of symptoms in depression:
  Vegetative
  Cognitive
  Impulse control
  Behavioral
  Physical (somatic)

and tried harder. The reality is that depression is an illness, not a choice, and is just as socially debilitating as coronary artery disease and more debilitating than diabetes mellitus or arthritis. Furthermore, up to 15% of severely depressed patients will ultimately commit suicide. Suicide attempts are up to ten per hundred subjects depressed for a year, with one successful suicide per hundred subjects depressed for a year. In the United States for example, there are approximately 300,000 suicide attempts and 30,000 suicides per year, most, but not all, associated with depression.

The conclusions are impressive: mood disorders are common, debilitating, life-threatening illnesses, which can be successfully treated but which commonly are not treated. Public education efforts are ongoing to identify cases and provide effective treatment.

Table 1–5. *Patient education*

The effectiveness of any treatment rests on a cooperative effort by patient and practitioner.
The patient should be told of the diagnosis, prognosis, and treatment options, including costs, duration, and potential side effects. In educating patient and family about the clinical management of depression, it is useful to emphasize the following information:
Depression is a medical illness, not a character defect or weakness.
Recovery is the rule, not the exception.
Treatments are effective, and there are many options for treatment. An effective treatment can be found for nearly all patients.
The aim of treatment is complete symptom remission, not just getting better but getting and staying well.
The risk of recurrence is significant: 50% after one episode, 70% after two episodes, 90% after three episodes.
Patient and family should be alert to early signs and symptoms of recurrence and seek treatment early if depression returns.

Table 1–6. *Risk factors for major depression*

Risk factor	Association
Sex	Major depresson is twice as likely in women
Age	Peak age on onset is 20–40 years
Family history	1.5 to 3 times higher risk with positive history
Marital status	Separated and divorced persons report higher rates
	Married males lower rates than unmarried males
	Married females higher rates than unmarried females
Postpartum	An increased risk for the 6-month period following childbirth
Negative life events	Possible association
Early parental death	Possible association

Table 1–7. *Depression in the United States*

High rate of occurence
    5–11% lifetime prevalence
    10–15 million in United States depressed in any year
Episodes can be of long duration (years)
Over 50% rate of recurrence following a single episode; higher if patient has had multiple episodes
Morbidity comparable to angina and advanced coronary artery disease
High mortality from suicide if untreated

Table 1–8. *Facts about suicide and depression*

20–40% of patients with an affective disorder exhibit nonfatal suicidal behaviors, including thoughts of suicide

Estimates associate 16,000 suicides in the United States annually with depressive disorder

15% of those hospitalized for major depressive disorder attempt suicide

15% of patients with severe primary major depressive disorder of at least 1 month's duration eventually commit suicide

Table 1–9. *Suicide and major depression: the rules of sevens*

One out of seven with recurrent depressive illness commits suicide

70% of suicides have depressive illness

70% of suicides see their primary care physician within 6 weeks of suicide

Suicide is the seventh leading cause of death in the United States

Table 1–10. *The hidden cost of not treating major depression*

Mortality
    30,000 to 35,000 suicides per year
    Fatal accidents due to impaired concentration and attention
    Death due to illnesses that can be sequelae (e.g., alcohol abuse)
Patient morbidity
    Suicide attempts
    Accidents
    Resultant illnesses
    Lost jobs
    Failure to advance in career and school
    Substance abuse
Societal costs
    Dysfunctional families
    Absenteeism
    Decreased productivity
    Job-related injuries
    Adverse effect on quality control in the workplace

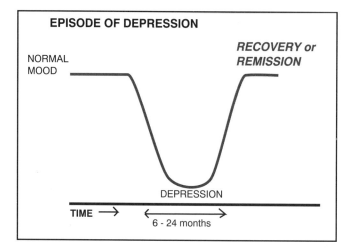

FIGURE 1–1. Depression is episodic, with **untreated episodes** commonly lasting 6 to 24 months, followed by **recovery** or **remission**.

Effects of Treatments on Mood Disorders

Long-Term Outcomes of Mood Disorders and the Five R's of Antidepressant Treatment

Until recently very little was really known about what happens to depression if it is not treated. It is now thought that most untreated episodes of depression last 6 to 24 months (Fig. 1–1). Perhaps only 5 to 10% of untreated sufferers have their episodes continue for more than 2 years. However, the very nature of this illness includes recurrent episodes. Many individuals who present for the first time for treatment will have a history of one or more prior unrecognized and untreated episodes of this illness, dating back to adolescence.

Three terms beginning with the letter "R" are used to describe the improvement of a depressed patient after treatment with an antidepressant, namely response, remission, and recovery. The term *response* generally means that a depressed patient has experienced at least a 50% reduction in symptoms as assessed on a standard psychiatric rating scale such as the Hamilton Depression Rating Scale (Fig. 1–2). This also generally corresponds to a global clinical rating of the patient as much improved or very much improved. *Remission*, on the other hand, is the term used when essentially all symptoms go away, not just 50% of them (Fig. 1–3). The patient is not better; the patient is actually well. If this lasts for 6 to 12 months, remission is then considered to be *recovery* (Fig. 1–3).

Two terms beginning with the letter "R" are used to describe worsening in a patient with depression, relapse and recurrence. If a patient worsens before there is a complete remission or before the remission has turned into a recovery, it is called a *relapse* (Fig. 1–4). However, if a patient worsens a few months after complete recovery, it is called a *recurrence*. The features that predict relapse with greatest accuracy are: (1) multiple prior episodes; (2) severe episodes; (3) long-lasting episodes; (4) episodes with bipolar or psychotic features; and (5) incomplete recovery between two consecutive episodes, also called poor interepisode recovery (Table 1–11).

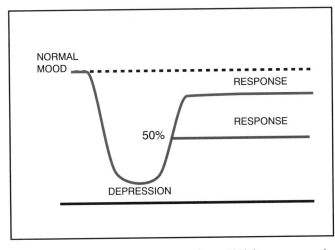

FIGURE 1–2. When treatment of depression results in at least 50% improvement in symptoms, it is called a **response**. Such patients are better, but not well.

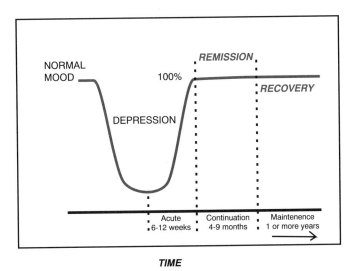

TIME

FIGURE 1–3. When treatment of depression results in removal of essentially all symptoms, it is called **remission** for the first several months, and then **recovery** if it is sustained for longer than 6 to 12 months. Such patients are not just better—they are well.

The longitudinal course of bipolar illness is also characterized by many recurrent episodes, some predominantly depressive, some predominantly manic or hypomanic, some mixed with simultaneous features of both mania and depression (Fig. 1–5); some may even be rapid cycling, with at least four ups and/or downs in 12 months (Fig. 1–6). There is worrisome evidence that bipolar disorders may be somewhat progressive, especially if uncontrolled. That is, mood fluctuations become more frequent, more severe, and less responsive to medications as time goes on, especially in cases where there has been little or inadequate treatment.

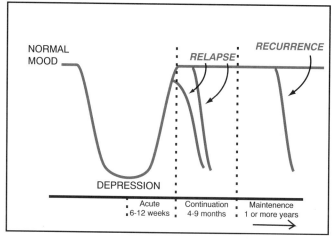

TIME

FIGURE 1–4. When depression returns before there is a full remission of symptoms or within the first several months following remission of symptoms, it is called a **relapse**. When depression returns after a patient has recovered, it is called a **recurrence**.

Table 1–11. *Biggest risk factors for a recurrent episode of depression*

Multiple prior episodes
Incomplete recoveries from prior episodes
Severe episode
Chronic episode
Bipolar or psychotic features

Dysthymia is a low-grade but very chronic form of depression, which lasts for more than 2 years (Fig. 1–7). It may represent a relatively stable and unremitting illness of low-grade depression, or it may indicate a state of partial recovery from an episode of major depressive disorder. When major depressive episodes are superimposed on dysthymia, the resulting condition is sometimes called "double depression" (Fig. 1–8) and may account for many of those with poor interepisode recovery.

Search for Subtypes of Depression That Predict Response to Antidepressants

Although effective for depression in general, antidepressants do not help everyone with depression. In fact, only about two out of three patients with depression will respond to any given antidepressant (Fig. 1–9), whereas only about one out of three will respond to placebo (Fig. 1–10). Follow-up studies of depressed patients after 1 year of clinical treatment show that approximately 40% still have the same diagnosis, 40% have no diagnosis, and the rest either recover partially or develop the diagnosis of dysthymia (Fig. 1–9). In the 1970s and 1980s, the diagnostic criteria

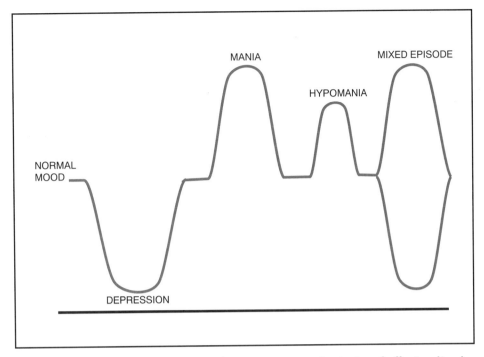

FIGURE 1–5. Bipolar disorder is characterized by various types of episodes of affective disorder, including **depression**, full **mania**, lesser degrees of mania called **hypomania**, and even **mixed episodes** in which mania and depression seem to coincide.

for depression began to focus in part on trying to identify those depressed patients who were the best candidates for the various antidepressant treatments that had become available.

During this era, the idea evolved that there might be one subgroup of unipolar depressives that was especially responsive to antidepressants and another that was not. The first group was hypothesized to have a serious, even melancholic clinical form of depression, which had a biological basis and a high degree of familial occurrence, was episodic in nature, and was likely to respond to tricyclic antidepressants and monoamine oxidase (MAO) inhibitors. Opposed to this was a second form of depression hypothesized to be neurotic and characterological in origin, less severe but more chronic, not especially responsive to antidepressants, and possibly amenable to treatment by psychotherapy. This was called depressive neurosis, or dysthymia.

The search for any biological markers of depression, let alone those that might be predictive of antidepressant treatment responsiveness has been disappointing. It is currently not possible to predict which patient will respond to antidepressants in general or to any specific antidepressant drug. However, it is well established that no matter what the subtype, some patients with any known form of unipolar depression will respond to antidepressants, including those individuals with melancholia as well as those with dysthymia.

Although it is therefore not yet possible to predict who will and who will not respond to a given antidepressant drug, several approaches that fail to predict this are known. These include the concepts of biological versus nonbiological, endogenous

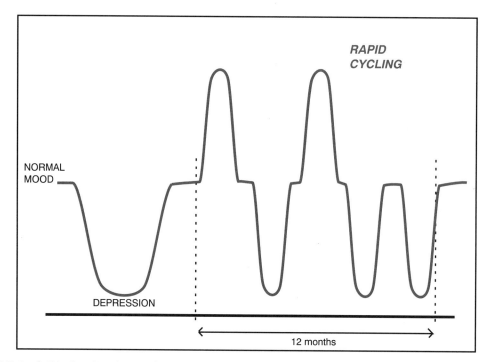

FIGURE 1–6. Bipolar disorder can become **rapid cycling**, with at least four switches into mania, hypomania, depression, or mixed episodes within a 12-month period. This is a particularly difficult form of bipolar disorder to treat.

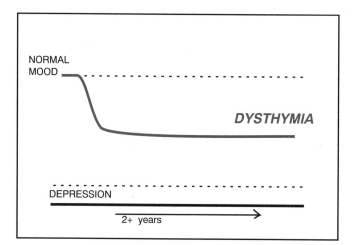

FIGURE 1–7. **Dysthymia** is a low-grade but very chronic form of depression, which lasts for more than 2 years.

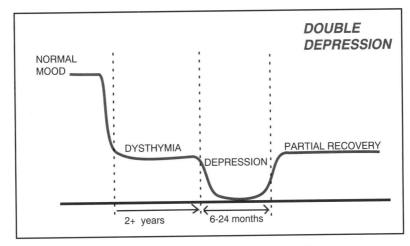

FIGURE 1−8. **Double depression** is a syndrome characterized by oscillation between episodes of major depression and periods of partial recovery or dysthymia.

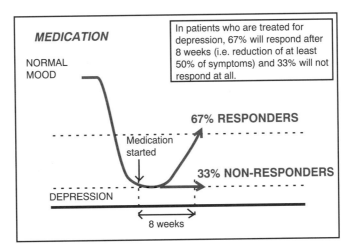

FIGURE 1−9. Virtually every known antidepressant has the same **response rate**, namely 67% of depressed patients respond to a given medication and 33% fail to respond.

versus reactive, melancholic versus neurotic, acute versus chronic, and familial versus nonfamilial depression, and others as well.

The Good News and the Bad News about Antidepressant Treatments

One can look at the effects of antidepressant treatments on the long-term outcome from depression as either good news or bad news, depending on whether it is seen from the perspective of *response* or from the perspective of *remission*. The news looks good if mere response to an antidepressant is the standard (i.e., getting better), but if one "raises the bar" and asks about remission (i.e., getting well), the news does not look nearly as good (Tables 1−12 and 1−13).

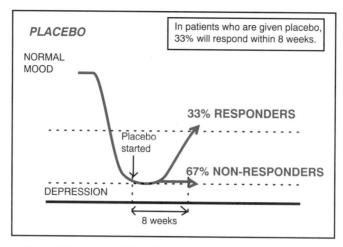

FIGURE 1–10. In controlled clinical trials, 33% of patients respond to **placebo** treatment and 67% fail to respond.

Table 1–12. *Limitations of response definition*

Response is a reduction in the signs and symptoms of depression of more than 50% from baseline.
Responders have residual symptoms.
Response is the end point for clinical trials, *not* clinical practice.

Table 1–13. *Remission*

Remission is defined as a Hamilton Depression Score less than 8 to 10 and a clinical global impression rating of normal, not mentally ill.
A patient who is in remission may be considered asymptomatic.
Remission is a more relevant end point than response for clinicians, as it signifies that the patient is "well."

For example, the good news side of the story is that half to two-thirds of patients respond to any given antidepressant, as mentioned above (Fig. 1–9 and Table 1–14). Even better news is the finding that 90% or more may eventually respond if a number of different antidepressants or combinations of antidepressants are tried in succession. Other good news is that some studies suggest that up to half of responders may go on to experience a complete remission from their depression within 6 months of treatment, and possibly two-thirds or more of the responders will remit within 2 years.

Some of the best news of all is that antidepressants significantly reduce relapse rates during the first 6 to 12 months following initial response to the medication (Figs. 1–11 and 1–12). That is, about half of patients may relapse within 6 months

Table 1–14. *The good news in the treatment of depression*

Half of depressed patients may recover within 6 months of an index episode of depression, and three-fourths may recover within 2 years.

Up to 90% of depressed patients may respond to one or a combination of therapeutic interventions if multiple therapies are tried.

Antidepressants reduce relapse rates.

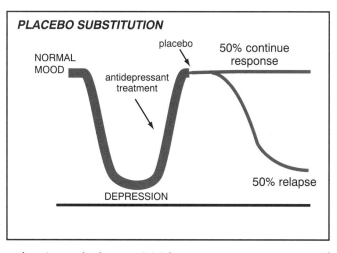

FIGURE 1–11. Depressed patients who have an initial treatment response to an antidepressant will **relapse at the rate of 50%** within 6 to 12 months if their medication is withdrawn and a **placebo substituted**.

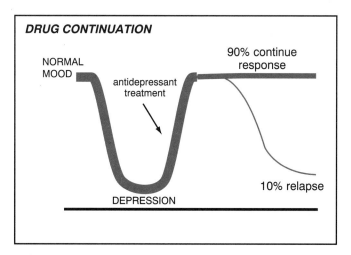

FIGURE 1–12. Depressed patients who have an initial treatment response to an antidepressant will **only relapse at the rate of about 10 to 20%** if their **medication is continued for a year** following recovery.

Table 1–15. *Probability of recurrence as a function of the number of previous episodes*

Number of Prior Episodes	Recurrence Risk
1	<50%
2	50–90%
3 or more	>90%

Table 1–16. *Who needs maintenance therapy?*

Patients with:
  Two or more prior episodes
  One prior episode (elderly, youth)
  Chronic episodes
  Incomplete remission

Table 1–17. *The bad news in the treatment of depression*

"Pooping out" is common: the percentage of patients who remain well during the 18-month period following successful treatment for depression is disappointingly low, only 70 to 80%.

Many patients are "treatment-refractory": the percentage of patients who are nonresponders and who have a very poor outcome during long-term follow-up evaluation after a diagnosis of depression is disappointingly high, up to 20%.

Up to half of patients may fail to attain remission, including both those with "apathetic" responses and those with "anxious" responses.

of response if they are switched to placebo (Fig. 1–11), but only about 10 to 25% relapse if they are continued on the drug that made them respond (Fig. 1–12).

On the basis of these findings, treatment guidelines have recently evolved so that depression is not just treated until a response is seen but treatment is continued after attaining a response, so that relapses are prevented (Tables 1–15 and 1–16). Those with their first episode of depression may need treatment for only 1 year following response, unless they had a very prolonged or severe episode, were elderly, were psychotic, or had a response but not a remission. Those with more than one episode may require lifelong treatment with an antidepressant, as the risk of relapse skyrockets the more episodes that a patient experiences (Tables 1–15 and 1–16). Antidepressant treatment reduces these relapse rates, especially in the first year after successful treatment (Figs. 1–11 and 1–12).

The bad news in the treatment of depression (Table 1–17) is that a common experience of antidepressant responders is that their treatment response will "poop out." That is, the percentage of patients who fail to maintain their response during the first 18 months following successful treatment for depression is disappointingly

Table 1–18. *Features of partial remission*

Apathetic responders:
  Reduction of depressed mood
  Continuing anhedonia, lack of motivation, decreased libido, lack of interest, no zest
  Cognitive slowing and decreased concentration
Anxious responders:
  Reduction of depressed mood
  Continuing anxiety, especially generalized anxiety
  Worry, insomnia, somatic symptoms

high, up to 20 to 30%. "Pooping out" may be even more likely in patients who only responded and never remitted (i.e., they never became well).

Although clinical trials conducted under ideal conditions for up to 1 year have high compliance and low dropout rates, this may not reflect what happens in actual clinical practice. Thus, the effectiveness of drugs (how well they work in the real world) may not approximate the efficacy of these same drugs (how well they work in clinical trials). For example, the median time of treatment with an antidepressant in clinical practice is currently only about 78 days, not 1 year, and certainly not a lifetime. Can you imagine treating hypertension or diabetes for only 78 days? Depression is a chronic, recurrent illness, which requires long-term treatment to maintain response and prevent relapses, just like hypertension and diabetes. Therefore, antidepressant *effectiveness* in reducing relapses in clinical practice will likely remain lower than antidepressant *efficacy* in clinical trials until long-term compliance can be increased.

Other bad news in the treatment of depression is that many responders never remit (Table 1–17). In fact, some studies suggest that up to half of patients who respond nevertheless fail to attain remission, including those with either "apathetic responses" or "anxious responses" (Table 1–18). The apathetic responder is one who experiences improved mood with treatment, but has continuing lack of pleasure (anhedonia), decreased libido, lack of energy, and no "zest." The anxious responder, on the other hand, is one who had anxiety mixed with depression and who experiences improved mood with treatment but has continuing anxiety, especially generalized anxiety characterized by excessive worry, plus insomnia and somatic symptoms. Both types of responders are better, but neither is well.

Why settle for silver when you can go for gold? Settling for mere response, whether apathetic or anxious, rather than pushing for full remission and wellness may be partly the fault of antidepressant prescribers, who have been taught that the end point for clinical research in journal publications and for approval by governmental regulatory agencies such as the U.S. Food and Drug Administration (FDA) is response, that is, a minimum of 50% improvement in symptoms (Table 1–12). Although response rates may be appropriate for research, remission rates are more relevant for clinical practice (Table 1–13). Responders may represent continuing illness in a milder form, as well as inadequate treatment, since matching the right antidepressant or combination of antidepressants to each patient will greatly increase the chance of delivering a full remission rather than a mere response (Table 1–19). Failure to push for remission means that the patient is left with an increased risk

Table 1–19. *Implications of partial response in patients who do not
attain remission*

Represents continuing illness in a milder form
Can be due to inadequate early treatment
Can also be due to underlying dysthymia or personality disorders
Leads to increased relapse rates
Causes continuing functional impairment
Associated with increased suicide rate

Table 1–20. *Dual mechanism hypothesis*

Remission rates are higher with antidepressants or with combinations of antidepressants
having dual serotonin and norepinephrine actions, as compared with those having
serotonin selective actions.
Corollary: Patients unresponsive to a single-action agent may respond, and eventually
remit, with dual-action strategies.

of relapse, continuing functional impairment, and a continuing increase in the risk
of suicide (Table 1–19). A patient who is in remission, on the other hand, may be
considered asymptomatic or well (Table 1–13).

Another bit of bad news is that many patients are treatment-refractory (Table
1–17). That is, the percentage of nonresponders with a very poor outcome is dis-
turbingly high—about 15 to 20% of all patients treated with antidepressants but
perhaps a majority of patients selectively referred to a modern psychiatrist's practice.

Fortunately, there is hope for eliminating the bad news stories listed here, namely
dual pharmacological mechanisms (Table 1–20). Data are increasingly showing that
the percentage of patients who remit is higher for antidepressants or combinations
of antidepressants acting synergistically on both serotonin and norepinephrine than
for those acting just on serotonin alone. Exploiting this strategy may help increase
the number of remitters, prevent or treat more cases of poop out, and convert treatment-refractory cases into successful outcomes. This will be discussed in more detail
in Chapter 3.

It is potentially important to treat symptoms of depression "until they are gone"
for reasons other than the obvious reduction of current suffering. Depression may
be part of an emerging theme for many psychiatric disorders today, namely, that
uncontrolled symptoms may indicate some ongoing pathophysiological mechanism
in the brain, which if allowed to persist untreated may cause the ultimate outcome
of illness to be worse. Depression seems to beget depression. Depression may thus
have a long-lasting or even irreversible neuropathological effect on the brain, ren-
dering treatment less effective if symptoms are allowed to progress than if they are
removed by appropriate treatment early in the course of the illness.

In summary, the natural history of depression indicates that this is a life-long
illness, which is likely to relapse within several months of an index episode, especially if untreated or under-treated or if antidepressants are discontinued, and is
prone to multiple recurrences that are possibly preventable by long-term antide-

pressant treatment. Antidepressant response rates are high, but remission rates are disappointingly low unless mere response is recognized and targeted for aggressive management, possibly by single drugs or combinations of drugs with dual serotonin-norepinephrine pharmacological mechanisms when selective agents are not fully effective.

Longitudinal Treatment of Bipolar Disorder

The mood stabilizer lithium was developed as the first treatment for bipolar disorder. It has definitely modified the long-term outcome of bipolar disorder because it not only treats acute episodes of mania, but it is the first psychotropic drug proven to have a prophylactic effect in preventing future episodes of illness. Lithium even treats depression in bipolar patients, although it is not so clear that it is a powerful antidepressant for unipolar depression. Nevertheless, it is used to augment antidepressants for treating resistant cases of unipolar depression.

Other mood stabilizers are arising from the group of drugs that were first developed as anticonvulsants and have also found an important place in the treatment of bipolar disorder. Several anticonvulsants are especially useful for the manic, mixed, and rapid cycling types of bipolar patients and perhaps for the depressive phase of this illness as well. Mood stabilizers will be discussed in detail in Chapter 3. Antipsychotics, especially the newer atypical antipsychotics, are also useful in the treatment of bipolar disorders.

Antidepressants modify the long-term course of bipolar disorder as well. When given with lithium or other mood stabilizers, they may reduce depressive episodes. Interestingly, however, antidepressants can flip a depressed bipolar patient into mania, into mixed mania with depression, or into chaotic rapid cycling every few days or hours, especially in the absence of mood stabilizers. Thus, many patients with bipolar disorders require clever mixing of mood stabilizers and antidepressants, or even avoidance of antidepressants, in order to attain the best outcome.

Without consistent long-term treatment, bipolar disorders are potentially very disruptive. Patients often experience a chronic and chaotic course, in and out of the hospital, with psychotic episodes and relapses. There is a significant concern that intermittent use of mood stabilizers, poor compliance, and increasing numbers of episodes will lead to even more episodes of bipolar disorder, and with less responsiveness to lithium. Thus, stabilizing bipolar disorders with mood stabilizers, atypical antipsychotics, and antidepressants is increasingly important not only in returning these patients to wellness but in preventing unfavorable long-term outcomes.

Mood Disorders Across the Life Cycle: When Do Antidepressants Start Working?

Children. Despite classical psychoanalytic notions suggesting that children do not become depressed, recent evidence is quite to the contrary. Unfortunately, very little controlled research has been done on the use of antidepressants to treat depression in children, so no antidepressant is currently approved for treatment of depression in children. However, many of the newer antidepressants have been extensively tested in children with other conditions. For example, some antidepressants are approved for the treatment of children with obsessive-compulsive disorder. Thus, the safety of some antidepressants is well established in children even if their efficacy for depression is not. Nevertheless, antidepressant treatment studies in children are in progress, and extensive anecdotal observations suggest that antidepressants, particularly the newer, safer ones (see Chapters 2 and 3), are in fact useful for treating depressed children. Changes in FDA regulations have extended patent lives for new drugs in the United States if such drugs are also approved to treat children. Thankfully, this is now providing incentives for doing the research necessary to prove the safety and efficacy of antidepressants to treat depression in children, a long neglected area of psychopharmacology.

Perhaps even more important in children is the issue of bipolar disorder. Mania and mixed mania have not only been greatly underdiagnosed in children in the past but also have been frequently misdiagnosed as attention deficit disorder and hyperactivity. Furthermore, bipolar disorder misdiagnosed as attention deficit disorder and treated with stimulants can produce the same chaos and rapid cycling state as antidepressants can in bipolar disorder. Thus, it is important to consider the diagnosis of bipolar disorder in children, especially those unresponsive or apparently worsened by stimulants and those who have a family member with bipolar disorder. These children may need their stimulants and antidepressants discontinued and treatment with mood stabilizers such as valproic acid or lithium initiated.

Adolescents. Documentation of the safety and efficacy of antidepressants and mood stabilizers is better for adolescents than for children, although not at the standard for adults. That is unfortunate, because mood disorders often have their onset in adolescence, especially in girls. Not only do mood disorders frequently begin after puberty, but children with onset of a mood disorder prior to puberty often experience an exacerbation in adolescence. Synaptic restructuring dramatically increases after age 6 and throughout adolescence. Onset of puberty also occurs at this time of the life cycle. Such events may explain the dramatic rise in the incidence of the onset of mood disorders, as well as the exacerbation of preexisting mood disorders, during adolescence.

Unfortunately, mood disorders are frequently not diagnosed in adolescents, especially if they are associated with delinquent antisocial behavior or drug abuse. This is indeed unfortunate, as the opportunity to stabilize the disorder early in its course and possibly even to prevent adverse long-term outcomes associated with lack of adequate treatment can be lost if mood disorders are not aggressively diagnosed and treated in adolescence. The modern psychopharmacologist should have a high index of suspicion and increased vigilance to the presence of a mood disorder in adolescents, because treatments may well be just as effective in adolescents as they are in adults and perhaps more critical to preserve normal development of the individual.

Biological Basis of Depression

Monoamine Hypothesis

The first major theory about the biological etiology of depression hypothesized that depression was due to a deficiency of monoamine neurotransmitters, notably norepinephrine (NE) and serotonin (5-hydroxytryptamine [5HT]) (Figs. 1–13 through

MONOAMINE HYPOTHESIS

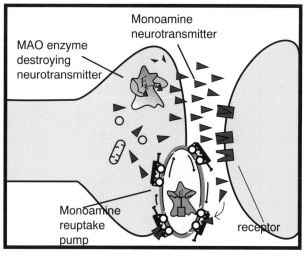

NORMAL STATE - NO DEPRESSION

FIGURE 1–13. This figure represents the **normal state** of a monoaminergic neuron. This particular neuron is releasing the neurotransmitter **norepinephrine (NE)** at the normal rate. All the regulatory elements of the neuron are also normal, including the functioning of the enzyme **monoamine oxidase (MAO), which destroys NE**, the **NE reuptake pump** which terminates the action of NE, and the **NE receptors** which react to the release of NE.

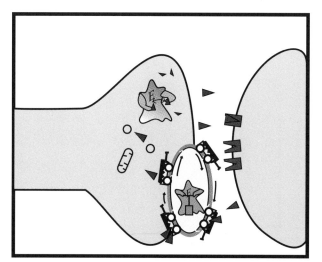

DEPRESSION: CAUSED BY NEUROTRANSMITTER DEFICIENCY

FIGURE 1–14. According to the monoamine hypothesis, in the case of **depression** the neurotransmitter is depleted, causing **neurotransmitter deficiency**.

21

MONOAMINE HYPOTHESIS

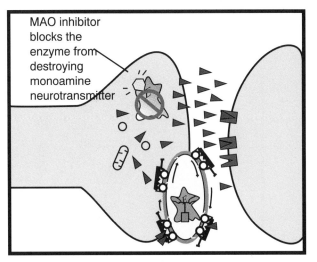

MAO inhibitor blocks the enzyme from destroying monoamine neurotransmitter

INCREASE IN NEUROTRANSMITTERS CAUSES RETURN TO NORMAL STATE

FIGURE 1–15. **Monoamine oxidase inhibitors** act as antidepressants, since they block the enzyme MAO from destroying monoamine neurotransmitters, thus allowing them to accumulate. This accumulation theoretically reverses the prior neurotransmitter deficiency (see Fig. 1–14) and according to the monoamine hypothesis, relieves depression by returning the monoamine neuron to the normal state.

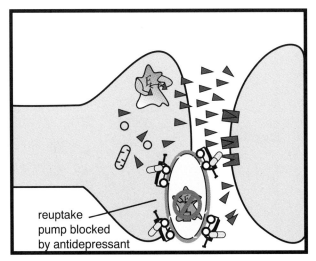

reuptake pump blocked by antidepressant

INCREASE IN NEUROTRANSMITTERS CAUSES RETURN TO NORMAL STATE

FIGURE 1–16. **Tricyclic antidepressants** exert their antidepressant action by blocking the neurotransmitter reuptake pump, thus causing neurotransmitter to accumulate. This accumulation, according to the monoamine hypothesis, reverses the prior neurotransmitter deficiency (see Fig. 1–14) and relieves depression by returning the monoamine neuron to the normal state.

1–16). Evidence for this was rather simplistic. Certain drugs that depleted these neurotransmitters could induce depression, and the known antidepressants at that time (the tricyclic antidepressants and the MAO inhibitors) both had pharmacological actions that boosted these neurotransmitters. Thus, the idea was that the "normal" amount of monoamine neurotransmitters (Fig. 1–13) became somehow depleted, perhaps by an unknown disease process, by stress, or by drugs (Fig. 1–14), leading to the symptoms of depression. The MAO inhibitors increased the monoamine neurotransmitters, causing relief of depression due to inhibition of MAO (Fig. 1–15). The tricyclic antidepressants also increased the monoamine neurotransmitters, resulting in relief from depression due to blockade of the monoamine transport pumps (Fig. 1–16). Although the monoamine hypothesis is obviously an overly simplified notion about depression, it has been very valuable in focusing attention on the three monoamine neurotransmitter systems norepinephrine, dopamine, and serotonin. This has led to a much better understanding of the physiological functioning of these three neurotransmitters and especially of the various mechanisms by which all known antidepressants act to boost neurotransmission at one or more of these three monoamine neurotransmitter systems.

Monoaminergic Neurons

In order to understand the monoamine hypothesis, it is necessary first to understand the normal physiological functioning of monoaminergic neurons. The principal monoamine neurotransmitters in the brain are the catecholamines norepinephrine (NE, also called noradrenaline) and dopamine (DA) and the indoleamine serotonin (5HT).

Noradrenergic neurons. The noradrenergic neuron uses NE for its neurotransmitter. Monoamine neurotransmitters are synthesized by means of enzymes, which assemble neurotransmitters in the cell body or nerve terminal. For the noradrenergic neuron, this process starts with tyrosine, the amino acid precursor of NE, which is transported into the nervous system from the blood by means of an active transport pump (Fig. 1–17). Once inside the neuron, the tyrosine is acted on by three enzymes in sequence, the first of which is tyrosine hydroxylase (TOH), the rate-limiting and most important enzyme in the regulation of NE synthesis. Tyrosine hydroxylase converts the amino acid tyrosine into dihydroxyphenylalanine (DOPA). The second enzyme DOPA decarboxylase (DDC), then acts, converting DOPA into dopamine (DA), which itself is a neurotransmitter in some neurons. However, for NE neurons, DA is just a precursor of NE. In fact, the third and final NE synthetic enzyme, dopamine beta-hydroxylase (DBH), converts DA into NE. The NE is then stored in synaptic packages called *vesicles* until released by a nerve impulse (Fig. 1–17).

Not only is NE created by enzymes, but it can also be destroyed by enzymes (Fig. 1–18). Two principal destructive enzymes act on NE to turn it into inactive metabolites. The first is MAO, which is located in mitochondria in the presynaptic neuron and elsewhere. The second is catechol-O-methyl transferase (COMT), which is thought to be located largely outside of the presynaptic nerve terminal (Fig. 1–18).

The action of NE can be terminated not only by enzymes that destroy NE, but also cleverly by a transport pump for NE, which removes it from acting in the synapse without destroying it (Fig. 1–18). In fact, such inactivated NE can be re-

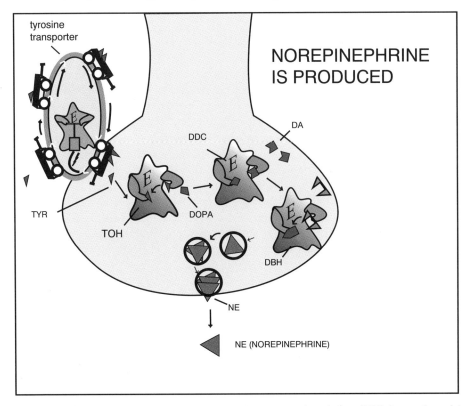

FIGURE 1–17. This figure shows how the neurotransmitter **norepinephrine (NE) is produced** in noradrenergic neurons. This process starts with the amino acid precursor of NE, **tyrosine (tyr)**, being transported into the nervous system from the blood by means of an active transport pump (tyrosine transporter). This active transport pump for tyrosine is separate and distinct from the active transport pump for NE itself (see Fig. 1–18). Once pumped inside the neuron, the tyrosine is acted on by three enzymes in sequence, the first of which, tyrosine hydroxylase (**TOH**), is the rate-limiting and most important enzyme in the regulation of NE synthesis. Tyrosine hydroxylase converts the amino acid tyrosine into **DOPA**. The second enzyme, namely DOPA decarboxylase (**DDC**), then acts by converting DOPA into dopamine (**DA**). The third and final NE synthetic enzyme, dopamine beta hydroxylase (**DBH**), converts DA into NE. The NE is then stored in synaptic packages called vesicles until released by a nerve impulse.

stored for reuse in a later neurotransmitting nerve impulse. The transport pump that terminates the synaptic action of NE is sometimes called the NE "transporter" and sometimes the NE "reuptake pump." This NE reuptake pump is located as part of the presynaptic machinery, where it acts as a vacuum cleaner, whisking NE out of the synapse and off the synaptic receptors and stopping its synaptic actions. Once inside the presynaptic nerve terminal, NE can either be stored again for subsequent reuse when another nerve impulse arrives, or it can be destroyed by NE-destroying enzymes (Fig. 1–18).

The noradrenergic neuron is regulated by a multiplicity of receptors for NE (Fig. 1–19). In the classical subtyping of NE receptors, they were classified as either alpha or beta, depending on their preference for a series of agonists and antagonists. Next, the NE receptors were subclassified into alpha 1 and alpha 2 as well as beta 1 and

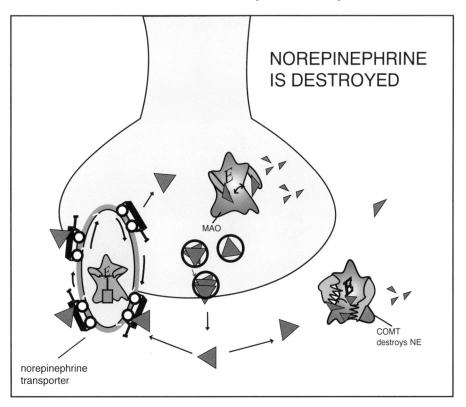

FIGURE 1–18. **Norepinephrine** (NE) can also be **destroyed** by enzymes in the NE neuron. The principal destructive enzymes are monoamine oxidase (**MAO**) and catechol-O-methyl transferase (**COMT**). The action of NE can be terminated not only by enzymes that destroy NE, but also by a transport pump for NE, called the **norepinephrine transporter**, which prevents NE from acting in the synapse without destroying it. This transport pump is separate and distinct from the transport pump for tyrosine used in carrying tyrosine into the NE neuron for NE synthesis (see Fig. 1–17). The transport pump that terminates the synaptic action of NE is sometimes called the "NE transporter" and sometimes the "NE reuptake pump." There are molecular differences among the transporters for the NE, dopamine, and serotonin neurons. These differences can be exploited by drugs so that the transport of one monoamine can be blocked independently of another. The NE transporter is part of the presynaptic machinery, where it acts as a "vacuum cleaner," whisking NE out of the synapse, and off the synaptic receptors and stopping its synaptic actions. Once inside the presynaptic nerve terminal, NE can either be stored again for subsequent reuse when another nerve impulse arrives, or it can be destroyed by enzymes.

beta 2. More recently, adrenergic receptors have been even further subclassified on the basis of both pharmacologic and molecular differences.

For a general understanding of NE receptors, the reader should begin with an awareness of three key receptors that are postsynaptic, namely beta 1, alpha 1, and alpha 2 receptors (Fig. 1–19). The postsynaptic receptors for NE convert occupancy of an alpha 1, alpha 2, or beta 1 receptor into a physiological function and ultimately result in changes in gene expression in the postsynaptic neuron.

On the other hand, alpha 2 receptors are the only presynaptic noradrenergic receptors on noradrenergic neurons. They regulate NE release and so are called *auto-receptors*. Presynaptic alpha 2 autoreceptors are located both on the axon terminal,

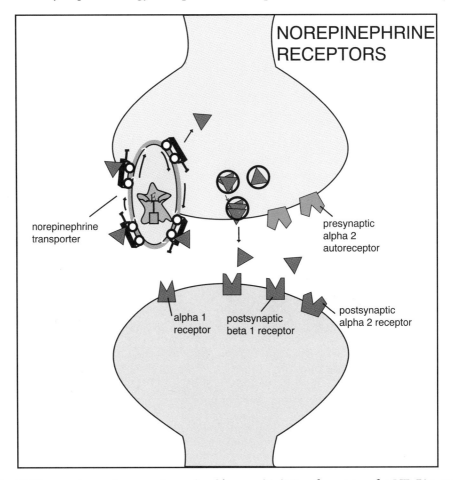

FIGURE 1–19. The noradrenergic neuron is regulated by a multiplicity of **receptors for NE**. Pictured here are the **NE transporter** and several NE receptors, including the presynaptic alpha 2 autoreceptor as well as the postsynaptic alpha 1, alpha 2 and beta 1 adrenergic receptors. The **presynaptic alpha 2 receptor** is important because it is an autoreceptor. That is, when the presynaptic alpha 2 receptor recognizes synaptic NE, it turns off further release of NE. Thus, the presynaptic alpha 2 terminal autoreceptor acts as a brake for the NE neuron. Stimulating this receptor (i.e., stepping on the brake) stops the neuron from firing. This probably occurs physiologically to prevent too much firing of the NE neuron, since it can shut itself off once the firing rate gets too high and the autoreceptor becomes stimulated. Postsynaptic NE receptors generally act by recognizing when NE is released from the presynaptic neuron and react by setting up a molecular cascade in the postsynaptic neuron, thereby causing neurotransmission to pass from the presynaptic to the postsynaptic neuron.

(terminal alpha 2 receptors) (Fig. 1–19) and at the cell body (soma) and nearby dendrites (somatodendritic alpha 2 receptors) (Fig. 1–20). Presynaptic alpha 2 receptors are important because both the terminal and the somatodendritic receptors are autoreceptors. That is, when presynaptic alpha 2 receptors recognize NE, they turn off further release of NE (Figs. 1–21 and 1–22). Thus, presynaptic alpha 2 autoreceptors act as a brake for the NE neuron and also cause what is known as a negative feedback regulatory signal. Stimulating this receptor (i.e., stepping on the brake) stops the neuron from firing. This probably occurs physiologically to prevent

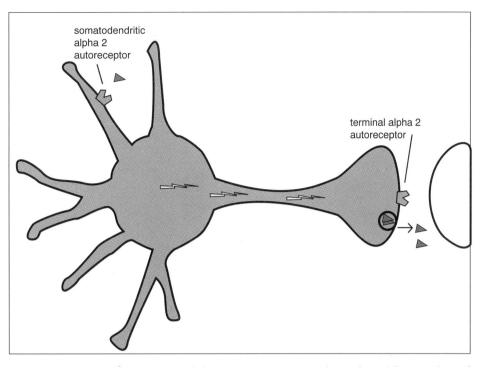

FIGURE 1–20. Both types of presynaptic alpha 2 autoreceptors are shown here. They are located either on the axon terminal, where they are called **terminal alpha 2 receptors**, or at the cell body (soma) and nearby dendrites, where they are called **somatodendritic alpha 2 receptors**.

overfiring of the NE neuron, since it can shut itself off once the firing rate gets too high and the autoreceptor becomes stimulated. It is worthy of note that not only can drugs mimic the natural functioning of the NE neuron by stimulating the presynaptic alpha 2 neuron, but drugs that antagonize this same receptor will have the effect of cutting the brake cable and enhancing the release of NE

Most of the cell bodies for noradrenergic neurons in the brain are located in the brainstem in an area known as the *locus coeruleus* (Fig. 1–23). The principal function of the locus coeruleus is to determine whether attention is being focused on the external environment or on monitoring the internal milieu of the body. It helps to prioritize competing incoming stimuli and fixes attention on just a few of these. Thus, one can either react to a threat from the environment or to signals such as pain coming from the body. Where one is paying attention will determine what one learns and what memories are formed as well.

Norepinephrine and the locus coeruleus are also thought to have an important input into the central nervous system's control of cognition, mood, emotions, movements, and blood pressure. Malfunction of the locus coeruleus is hypothesized to underlie disorders in which mood and cognition intersect, such as depression, anxiety, and disorders of attention and information processing. A norepinephrine deficiency syndrome (Table 1–21) is theoretically characterized by impaired attention, problems in concentrating, and difficulties specifically with working memory and the speed of information processing, as well as psychomotor retardation, fatigue, and

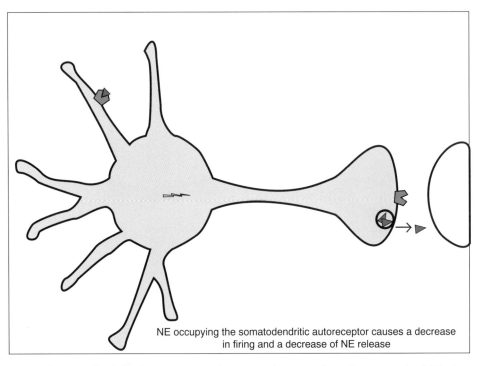

NE occupying the somatodendritic autoreceptor causes a decrease
in firing and a decrease of NE release

FIGURE 1–21. Presynaptic alpha 2 receptors are important because when they recognize NE, they turn off further release of NE. Shown here is the function of **presynaptic somatodendritic autoreceptors**, namely to act as a brake for the NE neuron and also to cause what is known as a negative feedback regulatory signal. Stimulating this receptor (i.e., "**stepping on the brake**") stops the neuron from firing. This probably occurs physiologically to prevent excessive firing of the NE neuron, since NE can shut itself off once the firing rate gets too high and the autoreceptor becomes stimulated.

apathy. Such symptoms can commonly accompany depression as well as other disorders with impaired attention and cognition, such as attention deficit disorder, schizophrenia, and Alzheimer's disease.

There are many specific noradrenergic pathways in the brain, each mediating a different physiological function. For example, one projection from the locus coeruleus to frontal cortex is thought to be responsible for the regulatory actions of NE on mood (Fig. 1–24); another projection to prefrontal cortex mediates the effects of NE on attention (Fig. 1–25). Different receptors may mediate these differential effects of norepinephrine in frontal cortex, postsynaptic beta 1 receptors for mood (Fig. 1–24) and postsynaptic alpha 2 for attention and cognition (Fig. 1–25).

The projection from the locus coeruleus to limbic cortex may regulate emotions, as well as energy, fatigue, and psychomotor agitation or psychomotor retardation (Fig. 1–26). A projection to the cerebellum may regulate motor movements, especially tremor (Fig. 1–27). Brainstem norepinephrine in cardiovascular centers controls blood pressure (Fig. 1–28). Norepinephrine from sympathetic neurons leaving the spinal cord to innervate peripheral tissues control heart rate (Fig. 1–29) and bladder emptying (Fig. 1–30).

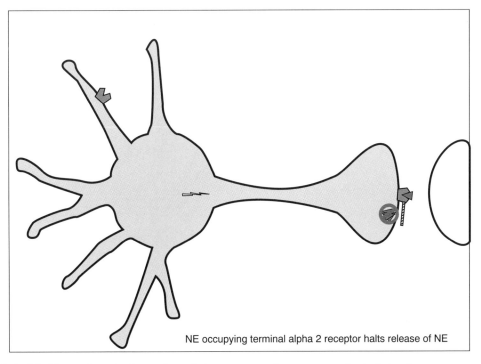

NE occupying terminal alpha 2 receptor halts release of NE

FIGURE 1–22. Shown here is the action of the **presynaptic axon terminal alpha 2 receptors,** which have the same function as the somatodendritic autoreceptors shown in Figure 1–21.

Dopaminergic neurons. Dopaminergic neurons utilize the neutotransmitter DA, which is synthesized in dopaminergic nerve terminals by two out of three of the same enzymes that also synthesize NE (Fig. 1–31). However, DA neurons lack the third enzyme, namely, dopamine beta hydroxylase, and thus cannot convert DA to NE. Therefore, it is DA that is stored and used for neurotransmitting purposes.

The DA neuron has a presynaptic transporter (reputake pump), which is unique for DA neurons (Fig. 1–32) but works analogously to the NE transporter (Fig. 1–33). On the other hand, the same enzymes that destroy NE (Fig. 1–18) also destroy DA (MAO and COMT) (Fig. 1–31).

Receptors for dopamine also regulate dopaminergic neurotransmission (Fig. 1–33). A plethora of dopamine receptors exist, including at least five pharmacological subtypes and several more molecular isoforms. Perhaps the most extensively investigated dopamine receptor is the dopamine 2 receptor, as it is stimulated by dopaminergic agonists for the treatment of Parkinson's disease and blocked by do-pamine antagonist antipsychotics for the treatment of schizophrenia. Dopamine 1, 2, 3, and 4 receptors are all blocked by some atypical antipsychotic drugs, but it is not clear to what extent dopamine 1, 3, or 4 receptors contribute to the clinical properties of these drugs. Dopamine receptors can be presynaptic, where they func-tion as autoreceptors. They provide negative feedback input, or a braking action on the release of dopamine from the presynaptic neuron. (Fig. 1–33).

Serotonergic neurons. Analogous enzymes, transport pumps, and receptors exist in the 5HT neuron (Figs. 1–34 through 1–42). For synthesis of serotonin in serotonergic

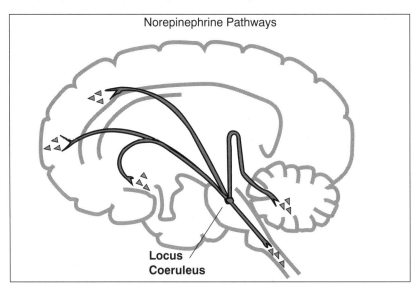

FIGURE 1–23. Most of the cell bodies for noradrenergic neurons in the brain are located in the brainstem in an area known as the **locus coeruleus**. This is the headquarters for most of the important noradrenergic pathways mediating behavior and other functions such as cognition, mood, emotions, and movements. Malfunction of the locus coeruleus is hypothesized to underlie disorders in which mood and cognition intersect, such as depression, anxiety, and disorders of attention and information processing.

Table 1–21. *Norepinephrine deficiency syndrome*

Impaired attention
Problems concentrating
Deficiencies in working memory
Slowness of information processing
Depressed mood
Psychomotor retardation
Fatigue

neurons, however, a different amino acid, tryptophan, is transported into the brain from the plasma to serve as the 5HT precursor (Fig. 1–34). Two synthetic enzymes then convert tryptophan into serotonin: first tryptophan hydroxylase converts tryptophan into 5-hydroxytryptophan, which is then converted by aromatic amino acid decarboxylase into 5HT (Fig. 1–34). Like NE and DA, 5HT is destroyed by MAO and converted into an inactive metabolite (Fig. 1–35). Also, the 5HT neuron has a presynaptic transport pump for serotonin called the serotonin transporter (Fig. 1–35), which is analogous to the NE transporter in NE neurons (Fig. 1–18) and to the DA transporter in DA neurons (Fig. 1–32).

Receptor subtyping for the serotonergic neuron has proceeded at a very rapid pace, with several major categories of 5HT receptors, each further subtyped

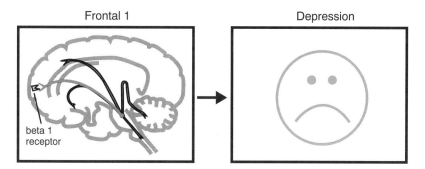

FIGURE 1–24. Some noradrenergic projections from the locus coeruleus to **frontal cortex** are thought to be responsible for the regulatory actions of norepinephrine on **mood**. **Beta 1** postsynaptic receptors may be important in transducing noradrenergic signals regulating mood in postsynaptic targets.

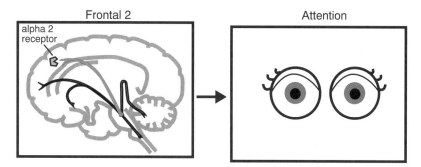

FIGURE 1–25. Other noradrenergic projections from the locus coeruleus to **frontal cortex** are thought to mediate the effects of norepinephrine on **attention**, concentration, and other **cognitive functions**, such as working memory and the speed of information processing. **Alpha 2** postsynaptic receptors may be important in transducing postsynaptic signals regulating attention in postsynaptic target neurons.

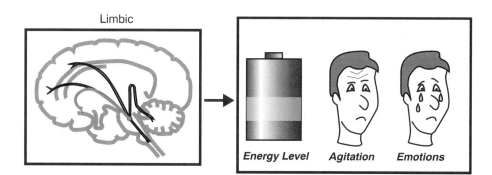

FIGURE 1–26. The noradrenergic projection from the locus coeruleus to **limbic cortex** may mediate emotions, as well as **energy**, fatigue, and psychomotor agitation or psychomotor retardation.

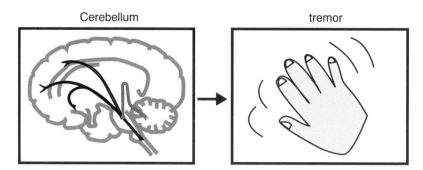

FIGURE 1–27. The noradrenergic projection from the locus coeruleus to the **cerebellum** may mediate motor movements, especially **tremor**.

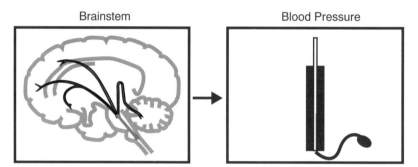

FIGURE 1–28. Brainstem norepinephrine in cardiovascular centers controls **blood pressure**.

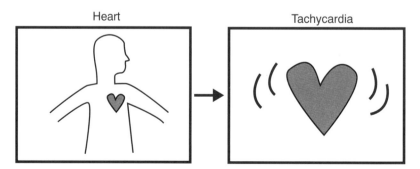

FIGURE 1–29. Noradrenergic innervation of the **heart** via sympathic neurons leaving the spinal cord regulates cardiovascular function, including **heart rate**, via beta 1 receptors.

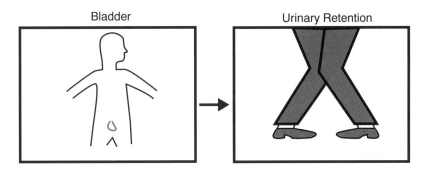

FIGURE 1–30. Noradrenergic innervation of the urinary tract via sympathetic neurons leaving the spinal cord regulates **bladder** emptying via alpha 1 receptors.

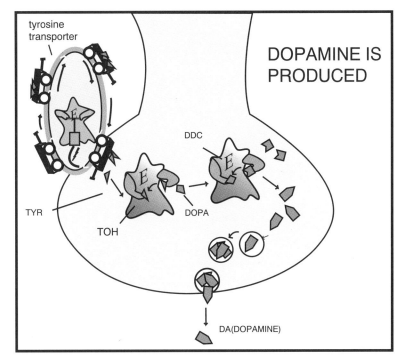

FIGURE 1–31. **Dopamine (DA)** is produced in dopaminergic neurons from the precursor **tyrosine (tyr)**, which is transported into the neuron by an active transport pump, called the tyrosine transporter, and then converted into DA by two of the same three enzymes that also synthesize norepinephrine (Fig. 1–17). The DA-synthesizing enzymes are tyrosine hydroxylase (**TOH**), which produces **DOPA**, and DOPA decarboxylase (**DDC**), which produces DA.

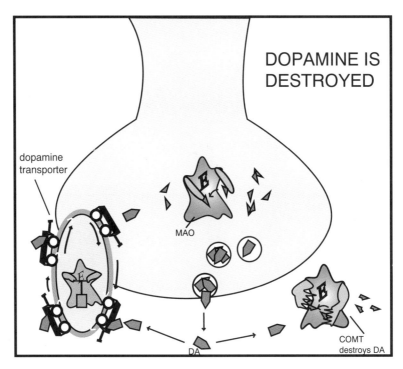

FIGURE 1–32. **Dopamine (DA)** is destroyed by the same enzymes that destroy norepinephrine (see Fig. 1–18), namely monoamine oxidase (**MAO**) and catechol-O-methyl-transferase (**COMT**). The DA neuron has a presynaptic transporter (**reuptake pump**), which is unique to the DA neuron but works analogously to the NE transporter (Fig. 1–18).

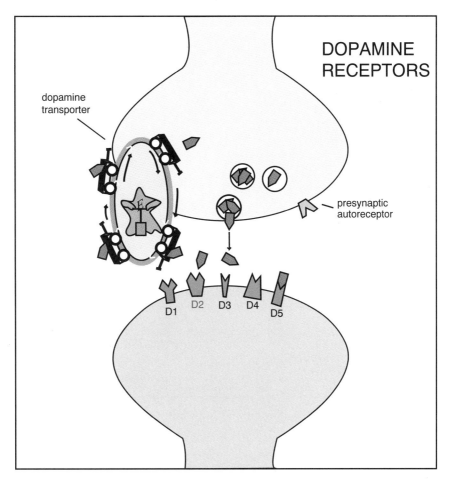

FIGURE 1–33. **Receptors for dopamine** (DA) regulate dopaminergic neurotransmission. A plethora of dopamine receptors exist, including at least five pharmacological subtypes and several more molecular isoforms. Perhaps the most extensively investigated dopamine receptor is the dopamine 2 (D2) receptor, as it is stimulated by dopaminergic agonists for the treatment of Parkinson's disease and blocked by dopamine antagonist neuroleptics and atypical antipsychotics for the treatment of schizophrenia.

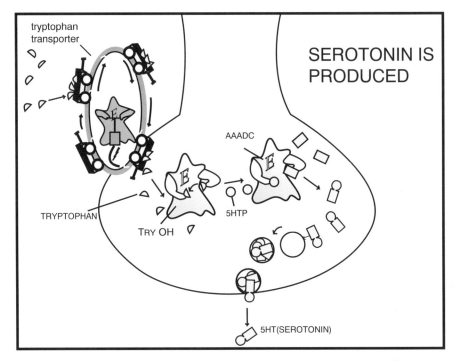

FIGURE 1–34. **Serotonin** (5-hydroxytryptamine [5HT]) is **produced** from enzymes after the amino acid precursor tryptophan is transported into the serotonin neuron. The **tryptophan transport pump** is distinct from the serotonin transporter (see Fig. 1–35). Once transported into the serotonin neuron, tryptophan is converted into 5-hydroxytryptophan (**5HTP**) by the enzyme tryptophan hydroxylase (**TryOH**) which is then converted into 5HT by the enzyme aromatic amino acid decarboxylase (**AAADC**). Serotonin is then stored in synaptic vesicles, where it stays until released by a neuronal impulse.

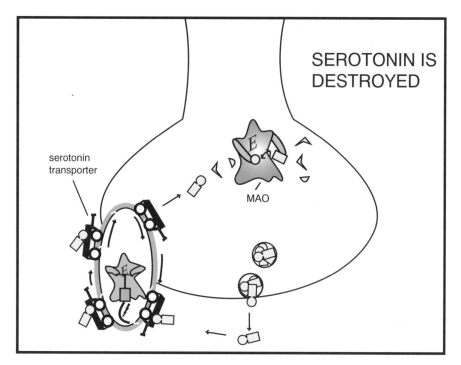

FIGURE 1–35. **Serotonin is destroyed** by the enzyme monoamine oxidase (**MAO**) and converted into an inactive metabolite. The 5HT neuron has a presynaptic transport pump selective for serotonin, which is called the **serotonin transporter** and is analogous to the norepinephrine (NE) transporter in NE neurons (Fig. 1–18) and to the DA transporter in DA neurons (Fig. 1–32).

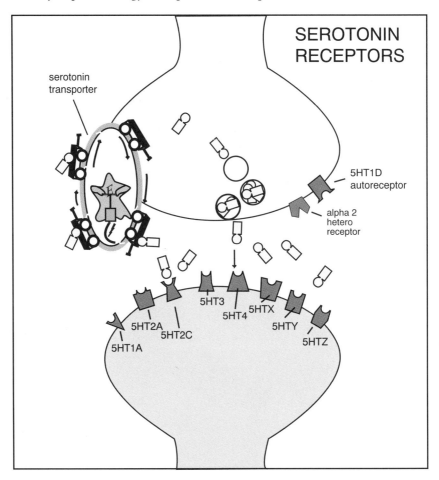

FIGURE 1–36. **Receptor subtyping for the serotonergic neuron** has proceeded at a very rapid pace, with at least four major categories of 5HT receptors, each further subtyped depending on pharmacological or molecular properties. In addition to the serotonin transporter, there is a key presynaptic serotonin receptor (the 5HT1D receptor) and another key presynaptic receptor, the alpha 2 noradrenergic heteroreceptor. This organization allows serotonin release to be controlled not only by serotonin but also by norepinephrine, even though the serotonin neuron does not itself release norepinephrine. Several postsynaptic serotonin receptors (5HT1A, 5HT1D, 5HT2A, 5HT2C, 5HT3, 5HT4, and many others denoted by 5HT X, Y, and Z) are shown as well. They convey messages from the presynaptic serotonergic neuron to the target cell postsynaptically.

depending on pharmacologic or molecular properties (Fig. 1–36). The 5HT receptors are a good example of how the description of neurotransmitter receptors is in constant flux and is constantly being revised. For a general understanding of the 5HT neuron, the reader can begin with an understanding that there are two key receptors that are presynaptic (5HT1A and 5HT1D) (Figs. 1–36 through 1–42) and several that are postsynaptic (5HT1A, 5HT1D, 5HT2A, 5HT2C, 5HT3, and 5HT4) (Fig. 1–36).

Presynaptic 5HT receptors are autoreceptors and detect the presence of 5HT, causing a shutdown of further 5HT release and 5HT neuronal impulse flow. When

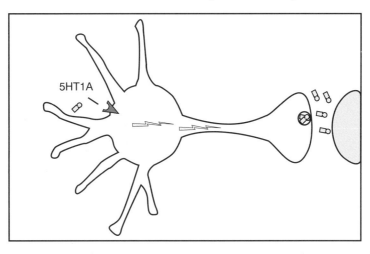

FIGURE 1–37. Presynaptic **5HT1A receptors** are autoreceptors, are located on the cell body and dendrites, and are therefore called somatodendritic autoreceptors.

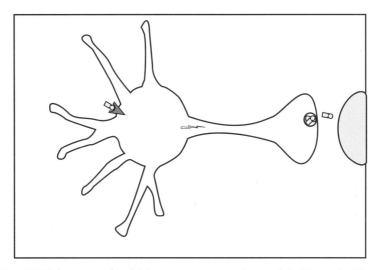

FIGURE 1–38. The **5HT1A somatodendritic autoreceptors** depicted in Figure 1–37 act by detecting the presence of 5HT and causing a **shutdown of 5HT neuronal impulse flow**, depicted here as decreased electrical activity and a reduction in the color of the neuron.

5HT is detected at the dendrites and cell body, this occurs via a 5HT1A receptor, which is also called a *somatodendritic* autoreceptor (Figs. 1–37 and 1–38). This causes a slowing of neuronal impulse flow through the serotonin neuron (Fig. 1–38). When 5HT is detected in the synapse by presynaptic 5HT receptors on axon terminals, this occurs via a 5HT1D receptor, also called a *terminal autoreceptor* (Fig. 1–39). In the case of the 5HT1D terminal autoreceptor, 5HT occupancy of this receptor inhibits 5HT release (Figs. 1–39 through 1–42). On the other hand, drugs that block the 5HT1D autoreceptor can promote 5HT release (Fig. 1–42).

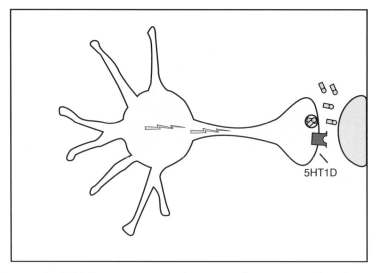

FIGURE 1–39. Presynaptic **5HT1D receptors** are also a type of autoreceptor, but they are located on the presynaptic axon terminal and are therefore called terminal autoreceptors.

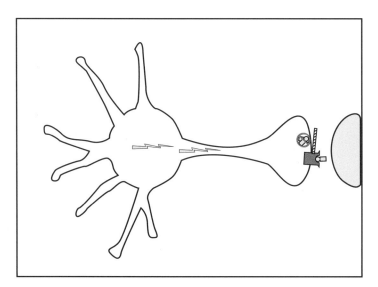

FIGURE 1–40. Depicted here is the consequence of the 5HT1D terminal autoreceptor being stimulated by serotonin. The terminal autoreceptor of Figure 1–39 is occupied here by 5HT, causing the **blockade of 5HT release**, as also shown in Fig. 1–41.

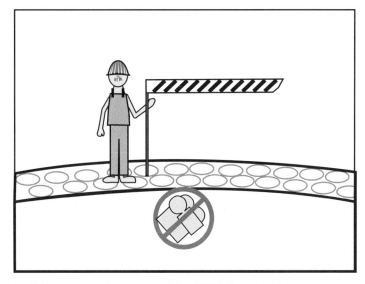

FIGURE 1–41. Depicted here is an enlargement of the 5HT1D terminal autoreceptor being stimulated by serotonin. The terminal autoreceptor of Figure 1–40 is occupied here by 5HT, causing the **blockade of 5HT release**.

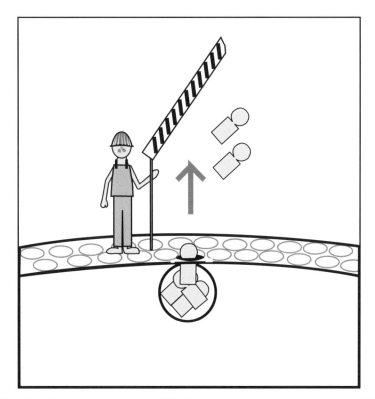

FIGURE 1–42. If a drug blocks a presynaptic **5HT1D terminal autoreceptor**, it would promote the release of 5HT by not allowing 5HT to block its own release. Some 5HT1D antagonists are being tested for the treatment of depression.

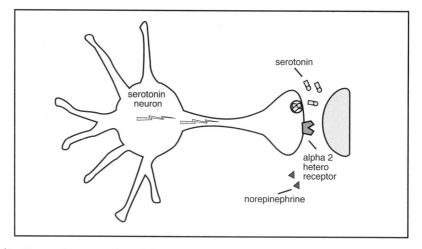

FIGURE 1—43. Shown here are the **alpha 2 presynaptic heteroreceptors** on serotonin axon terminals.

The serotonin neuron not only has serotonin receptors located presynaptically, but also has presynaptic noradrenergic receptors that regulate serotonin release (Figs. 1—36 and 1—43 through 1—46). On the axon terminal of serotonergic receptors are located presynaptic alpha 2 receptors (Figs. 1—35, 1—42, and 1—43), just as they are on noradrenergic neurons (Figs. 1—19 through 1—22). When norepinephrine is released from nearby noradrenergic neurons, it can diffuse to alpha 2 receptors, not only to those on noradrenergic neurons but also to the same receptors on serotonin neurons. Like its actions on noradrenergic neurons, norepinephrine occupancy of alpha 2 receptors on serotonin neurons will turn off serotonin release. Thus, serotonin release can be inhibited by serotonin and by norepinephrine. Alpha 2 receptors on a norepinephrine neuron are called *autoreceptors*, but alpha 2 receptors on serotonin neurons are called *heteroreceptors*.

Another type of presynaptic norepinephrine receptor on serotonin neurons is the alpha 1 receptor, located on the cell bodies (Figs. 1—45 and 1—46). When norepinephrine interacts with this receptor, it *enhances* serotonin release. Thus, norepinephrine can act as both an accelerator and a brake for serotonin release (Table 1—22 and Figs. 1—47 and 1—48).

The anatomic sites of noradrenergic control of serotonin release are shown in Figure 1—47, and include the "brake" at the axon terminals in the cortex and the "accelerator" at the cell bodies in the brainstem. This is shown schematically in Figure 1—48.

Postsynaptic 5HT receptors such as 5HT2A receptors (Fig. 1—49) regulate the translation of 5HT release from the presynaptic nerve into a neurotransmission in the postsynaptic nerve (Fig. 1—50). The 5HT2A, 5HT2C, and 5HT3 receptors are especially important postsynaptic 5HT receptor subtypes because they are implicated in the several physiological actions of serotonin in various serotonin pathways in the central nervous system. More is being learned about the importance of postsynaptic 5HT1A receptors in the brain and 5HT4 receptors in the gastrointestinal tract.

The headquarters for the cell bodies of serotonergic neurons is in the brainstem area called the *raphe nucleus* (Fig. 1—51). Projections from the raphe to the frontal

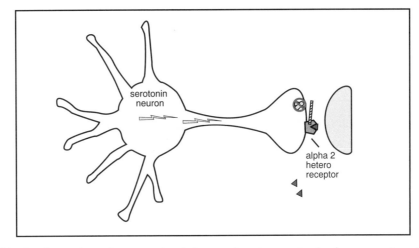

FIGURE 1–44. This figure shows how norepinephrine can function as a **brake for serotonin release**. When norepinephrine is released from nearby noradrenergic neurons, it can diffuse to alpha 2 receptors, not only to those on noradrenergic neurons but as shown here, also to these same receptors on serotonin neurons. Like its actions on noradrenergic neurons, norepinephrine occupancy of alpha 2 receptors on serotonin neurons will turn off serotonin release. Thus, serotonin release can be inhibited not only by serotonin but, as shown here, also by norepinephrine. Alpha 2 receptors on a norepinephrine neuron are called autoreceptors, but alpha 2 receptors on serotonin neurons are called **heteroreceptors**.

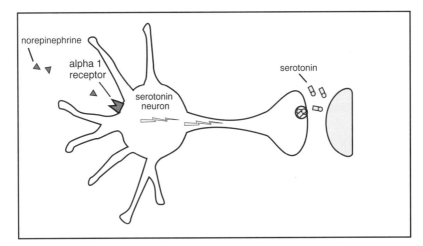

FIGURE 1–45. Another type of presynaptic norepinephrine receptor on serotonin neurons is the **alpha 1 receptor**, located on the cell bodies and dentrites.

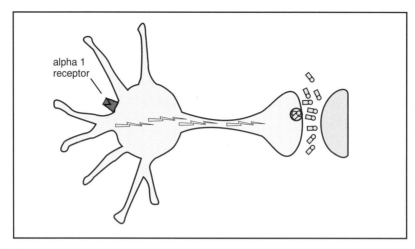

FIGURE 1–46. Shown here is how norepinephrine can act as a facilitator or "**accelerator**" of serotonin release. When norepinephrine interacts with the somatodendritic alpha 1 receptor on serotonin neurons, it enhances serotonin release.

Table 1–22. *Types of noradrenergic interactions with serotonin*

Inhibitory
Axoaxonic interactions (noradrenergic axons with serotonergic axon terminals)
Inhibitory alpha 2 heteroreceptors (negative feedback)
"Brakes"
Excitatory
Axodendritic interactions (noradrenergic axons with serotonergic cell bodies and dendrites)
Excitatory alpha 1 receptors (positive feedback)
"Accelerators"

cortex may be important for regulating mood (Fig. 1–52). Projections to basal ganglia, especially on 5HT2A receptors, may help control movements and obsessions and compulsions (Fig. 1–53). Projections from the raphe to the limbic area, especially on 5HT2A and 5HT2C postsynaptic receptors, may be involved in anxiety and panic (Fig. 1–54). Projections to the hypothalamus especially on 5HT3 receptors may regulate appetite and eating behavior (Fig. 1–55). Brainstem sleep centers, especially with 5HT2A postsynaptic receptors, regulate sleep, especially slow-wave sleep (Fig. 1–56). Serotonergic neurons descending down the spinal cord may be responsible for controlling certain spinal reflexes that are part of the sexual response, such as orgasm and ejaculation (Fig. 1–57). The brainstem chemoreceptor trigger zone can mediate vomiting, especially via 5HT3 receptors (Fig. 1–58). Peripheral 5HT3 and 5HT4 receptors may also regulate appetite as well as other gastrointestinal functions, such as gastrointestinal motility (Fig. 1–59). Putting all these pathways and their functions together, a hypothetical serotonin deficiency syndrome (Table 1–23) might comprise depression, anxiety, panic, phobias, obsessions, compulsions, and food craving.

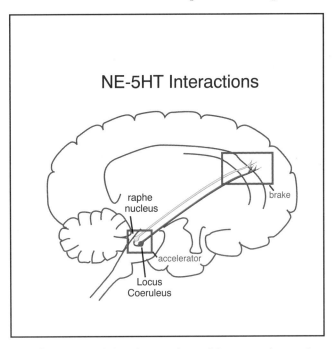

FIGURE 1–47. Two types of **norepinephrine interaction with serotonin** are shown here. In the brainstem, a pathway from locus coeruleus to raphe interacts with serotonergic cell bodies there and **accelerates** serotonin release. A second noradrenergic pathway to target areas in the cortex also interacts with serotonin axon terminals there and **brakes** serotonin release.

Classical Antidepressants and the Monoamine Hypothesis

The first antidepressants to be discovered came from two classes of agents, namely, the tricyclic antidepressants, so named because their chemical structure has three rings, and the MAO inhibitors, so named because they inhibit the enzyme MAO, which destroys monoamine neurotransmitters. When tricyclic antidepressants block the NE transporter, they increase the availability of NE in the synapse, since the "vacuum cleaner" reuptake pump can no longer sweep NE out of the synapse (Figs. 1–16 and 1–18). When tricyclic antidepressants block the DA pump (Fig. 1–32) or the 5HT pump (Fig. 1–35), they similarly enhance the synaptic availability of DA or 5HT, respectively, and by the same mechanism. When MAO inhibitors block NE, DA, and 5HT breakdown, they boost the levels of these neurotransmitters (Fig. 1–15).

Since it was recognized by the 1960s that all the classical antidepressants boost NE, DA, and 5HT in one manner or another (Figs. 1–15 and 1–16), the original idea was that one or another of these neurotransmitters, also chemically known as monoamines, might be deficient in the first place in depression (Fig. 1–14). Thus, the "monoamine hypothesis" was born. A good deal of effort was expended, especially in the 1960s and 1970s, to identify the theoretically predicted deficiencies of the monoamine neurotransmitters. This effort to date has unfortunately yielded mixed and sometimes confusing results.

Some studies suggest that NE metabolites are deficient in some patients with depression, but this has not been uniformly observed. Other studies suggest that

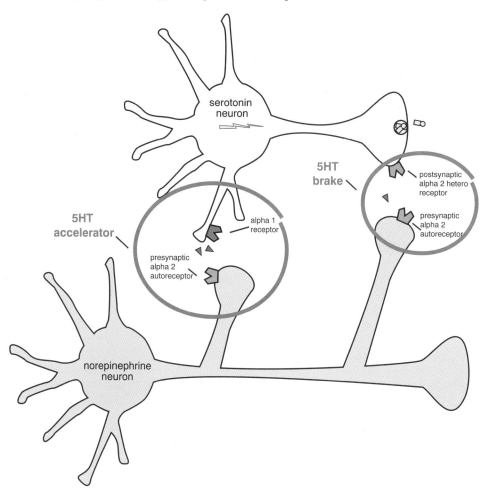

FIGURE 1–48. A schematic representation of both the **excitatory and inhibitory actions of norepinephrine on serotonin release** is shown here. This is the same action shown in Figure 1–47.

the 5HT metabolite 5-hydroxy-indole acetic acid (5HIAA) is reduced in the cerebrospinal fluid (CSF) of depressed patients. On closer examination, however, it has been found that only some of the depressed patients have low CSF 5HIAA, and these tend to be the patients with impulsive behaviors, such as suicide attempts of a violent nature. Subsequently, it was also reported that CSF 5HIAA is decreased in other populations who were subject to violent outbursts of poor impulse control but were not depressed, namely, patients with antisocial personality disorder who were arsonists, and patients with borderline personality disorder with self-destructive behaviors. Thus, low CSF 5HIAA may be linked more closely with impulse control problems than with depression.

Another problem with the monoamine hypothesis is the fact that the timing of antidepressant effects on neurotransmitters is far different from the timing of the antidepressant effects on mood. That is, antidepressants boost monoamines *immedi-*

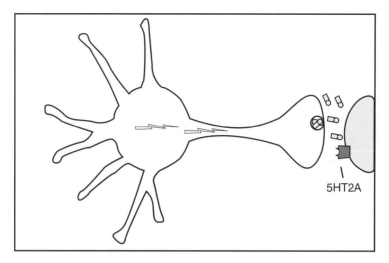

FIGURE 1–49. A key postsynaptic regulatory receptor is the **5HT2A receptor**.

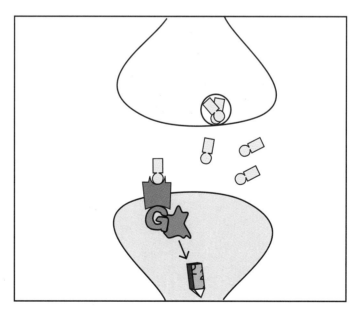

FIGURE 1–50. When the **postsynaptic 5HT2A receptor** of Figure 1–49 is occupied by 5HT, it causes neuronal impulses in the postsynaptic neuron to be transduced via the production of **second messengers**.

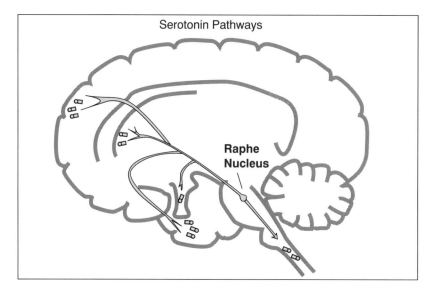

FIGURE 1–51. The headquarters for the cell bodies of serotonergic neurons is in the brainstem area called the **raphe nucleus**.

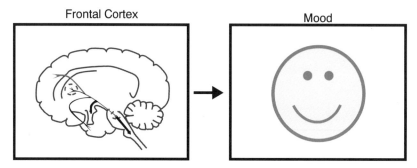

FIGURE 1–52. Serotonergic projections from raphe to **frontal cortex** may be important for regulating **mood**.

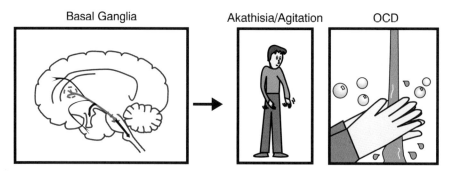

FIGURE 1–53. Serotonergic projections from raphe to **basal ganglia** may help control movements as well as **obsessions and compulsions**.

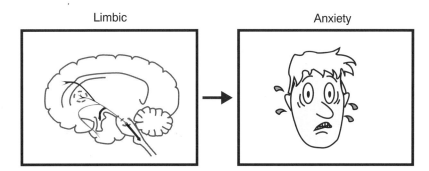

FIGURE 1–54. Serotonergic projections from raphe to **limbic** areas may be involved in **anxiety** and panic.

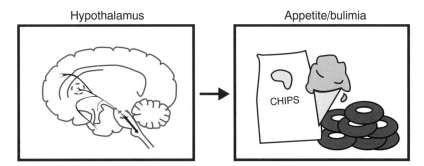

FIGURE 1–55. Serotonergic projections to the **hypothalamus** may regulate appetite and **eating** behavior.

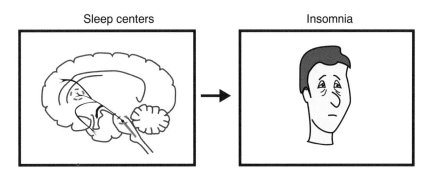

FIGURE 1–56. Serotonergic neurons in brainstem **sleep centers** regulate sleep, especially slow-wave sleep.

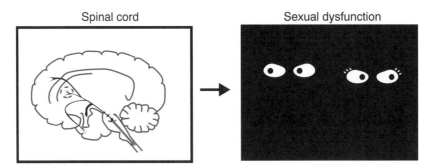

FIGURE 1–57. Serotonergic neurons descending down the **spinal cord** may be responsible for controlling certain spinal reflexes that are part of the **sexual response**, such as orgasm and ejaculation.

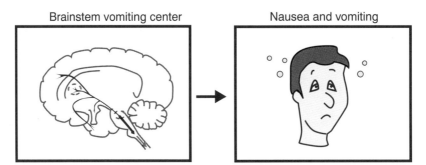

FIGURE 1–58. The chemoreceptor trigger zone in the **brainstem** can mediate **vomiting**, especially via 5HT3 receptors.

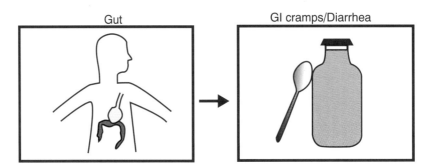

FIGURE 1–59. Peripheral 5HT3 and 5HT4 receptors in the **gut** may regulate appetite as well as other **gastrointestinal functions**, such as gastrointestinal motility.

Table 1–23. *Serotonin deficiency syndrome*

Depressed mood
Anxiety
Panic
Phobia
Anxiety
Obsessions and compulsions
Food craving; bulimia

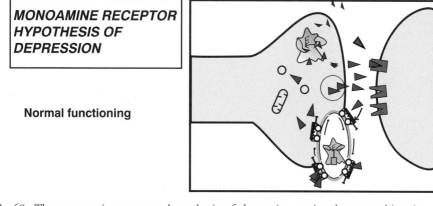

MONOAMINE RECEPTOR HYPOTHESIS OF DEPRESSION

Normal functioning

FIGURE 1–60. The monoamine receptor hypothesis of depression posits that something is wrong with the receptors for the key monoamine neurotransmitters. Thus, according to this theory, an abnormality in the receptors for monoamine neurotransmitters leads to depression. Such a disturbance in neurotransmitter receptors may be caused by depletion of monoamine neurotransmitters, by abnormalities in the receptors themselves, or by some problem with signal transduction of the neurotransmitter's message from the receptor to other downstream events. Depicted here is the **normal monoamine neuron** with the normal amount of monoamine neurotransmitter and the normal amount of correctly functioning monoamine receptors.

ately, but as mentioned earlier, there is a significant *delay* in the onset of their therapeutic actions, which in fact occurs many days to weeks *after* they have already boosted the monoamines. Because of these and other difficulties, the focus of hypotheses for the etiology of depression began to shift from the monoamine neurotransmitters themselves to their receptors. As we shall see, contemporary theories have shifted past the receptors to the molecular events that regulate gene expression.

Neurotransmitter Receptor Hypothesis

The neurotransmitter receptor theory posits that something is wrong with the receptors for the key monoamine neurotransmitters (Figs. 1–60 through 1–62). According to this theory, an abnormality in the receptors for monoamine neurotransmitters leads to depression (Fig. 1–62). Such a disturbance in neurotransmitter receptors may itself be caused by depletion of monoamine neurotransmitters (Fig. 1–61).

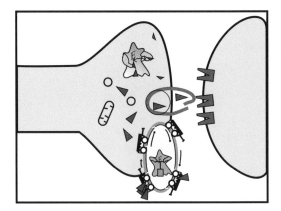

Decrease in NT

FIGURE 1–61. In this figure, **monoamine neurotransmitter is depleted** (see red circle), just as previously shown in Figure 1–14.

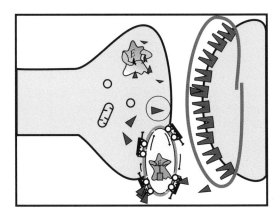

Receptors up-regulate due to lack of NT

FIGURE 1–62. The consequences of monoamine neurotransmitter depletion, of stress, or of some inherited abnormality in neurotransmitter receptor could cause the **postsynaptic receptors to abnormally up-regulate** (indicated in red circle). This up-regulation or other receptor dysfunction is hypothetically linked to the cause of depression.

Depletion of monoamine neurotransmitters (cf. Fig. 1–60 and Fig. 1–61) has already been discussed as the central theme of the monoamine hypothesis of depression (see Figs. 1–13 and 1–14). The neurotransmitter receptor hypothesis of depression takes this theme one step further—namely, that the depletion of neurotransmitter causes compensatory up regulation of postsynaptic neurotransmitter receptors (Fig. 1–62).

Direct evidence of this is generally lacking, but postmortem studies do consistently show increased numbers of serotonin 2 receptors in the frontal cortex of patients who commit suicide. Indirect studies of neurotransmitter receptor functioning in patients with major depressive disorders suggest abnormalities in various neurotransmitter receptors when using neuroendocrine probes or peripheral tissues such as platelets or lymphocytes. Modern molecular techniques are exploring for abnormalities in gene expression of neurotransmitter receptors and enzymes in families with depression but have not yet been successful in identifying molecular lesions.

The Monoamine Hypothesis of Gene Expression

So far, there is no clear and convincing evidence that monoamine deficiency accounts for depression; that is, there is no "real" monoamine deficit. Likewise, there is no clear and convincing evidence that excesses or deficiencies of monoamine receptors account for depression; that is, there is no pseudomonoamine deficiency due to the monoamines being there but not the monoamine receptors. On the other hand, there is growing evidence that despite apparently normal levels of monoamines and their receptors, these systems do not respond normally. For instance, probing monoaminergic receptors with drugs that stimulate them can lead to deficient output of neuroendocrine hormones. It can also lead to deficient changes in neuronal firing rates, as demonstrated on positron emission tomography (PET).

Such observations have led to the idea that depression may be a pseudomonoamine deficiency due to a deficiency in signal transduction from the monoamine neurotransmitter to its postsynaptic neuron in the presence of normal amounts of neurotransmitter and receptor. If there is a deficiency in the molecular events that cascade from receptor occupancy by neurotransmitter, it could lead to a deficient cellular response and thus be a form of pseudomonoamine deficiency (i.e., the receptor and the neurotransmitter are normal, but the transduction of the signal from neurotransmitter to its receptor is somehow flawed). Such a deficiency in molecular functioning has been described for certain endocrine diseases such as hypoparathyroidism (parathyroid hormone deficiency), pseudohypoparathyroidism (parathyroid receptors deficient but parathyroid hormone levels normal), and pseudo-pseudohypoparathyroidism (signal transduction deficiency leading to hypoparathyroid clinical state despite normal levels of hormone and receptor).

Perhaps a similar situation exists for depression due to a hypothesized problem within the molecular events distal to the receptor. Thus, second messenger systems leading to the formation of intracellular transcription factors that control gene regulation could be the site of deficient functioning of monoamine systems. This is the subject of much current research into the potential molecular basis of affective disorders. This hypothesis suggests some form of molecularly mediated deficiency in monoamines that is distal to the monoamines themselves and their receptors despite apparently normal levels of monoamines and numbers of monoamine receptors.

One candidate mechanism that has been proposed as the site of a possible flaw in signal transduction from monoamine receptors is the target gene for brain-derived neurotrophic factor (BDNF). Normally, BDNF sustains the viability of brain neurons, but under stress, the gene for BDNF is repressed (Fig. 1–63), leading to the atrophy and possible apoptosis of vulnerable neurons in the hippocampus when their BDNF is cut off (Fig. 1–64). This in turn leads to depression and to the consequences of repeated depressive episodes, namely, more and more episodes and less and less responsiveness to treatment. This possibility that hippocampal neurons are decreased in size and impaired in function during depression is supported by recent clinical imaging studies showing decreased brain volume of related structures. This provides a molecular and cellular hypothesis of depression consistent with a mechanism distal to the neurotransmitter receptor and involving an abnormality in gene expression. Thus, stress-induced vulnerability decreases the expression of genes that make neurotrophic factors such as BDNF critical to the survival and function of key neurons (Fig. 1–63). A corollary to this hypothesis is that antidepressants act to

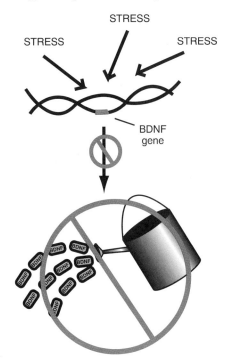

FIGURE 1–63. The monoamine hypothesis of gene action in depression, part 1. One candidate mechanism that has been proposed as the site of a possible flaw in signal transduction from monoamine receptors is the target gene for **brain-derived neurotrophic factor** (BDNF). Normally, BDNF sustains the viability of brain neurons. Shown here, however, is the gene for BDNF under situations of stress. In this case, the gene for BDNF is repressed, and BDNF is not being synthesized.

reverse this by causing the genes for neurotrophic factors to be activated (see Chapter 2).

Neurokinin Hypothesis of Emotional Dysfunction

Another hypothesis for the pathophysiology of depression and other states of emotional dysfunction relates to the actions of a relatively new class of peptide neurotransmitters known as *neurokinins* (also sometimes called *tachykinins*). This hypothesis was generated by some rather serendipitous observations that an antagonist to one of the neurokinins, namely substance P, may have antidepressant actions. Classically, substance P was thought to be involved in the pain response because it is released from neurons in peripheral tissues in response to inflammation, causing "neurogenic" inflammation and pain (Fig. 1–65). Furthermore, substance P is present in spinal pain pathways, suggesting a role in central nervous system-mediated pain (Fig. 1–65). Unfortunately, however, antagonists to substance P's receptors have so far been unable to reduce neurogenic inflammation or pain of many types in human testing.

On the other hand, suggestions that substance P antagonists may have improved mood, if not pain, in migraine patients led to controlled trials of such drugs in patients with depression. Although these are still early days and not all studies confirm antidepressant effects of substance P antagonists, the possibility that such

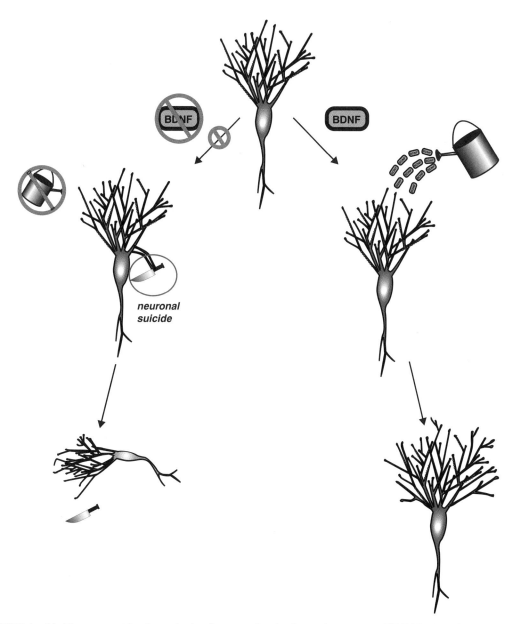

FIGURE 1−64. The monoamine hypothesis of gene action in depression, part 2. If BDNF is no longer made in appropriate amounts, instead of the neuron prospering and developing more and more synapses (right), **stress** causes vulnerable neurons in the hippocampus to **atrophy** and possibly undergo **apoptosis** when their neurotrophic factor is cut off (left). This, in turn, leads to depression and to the consequences of repeated depressive episodes, namely, more and more episodes and less and less responsiveness to treatment. This may explain why hippocampal neurons seem to be decreased in size and impaired in function during depression on the basis of recent clinical neuroimaging studies.

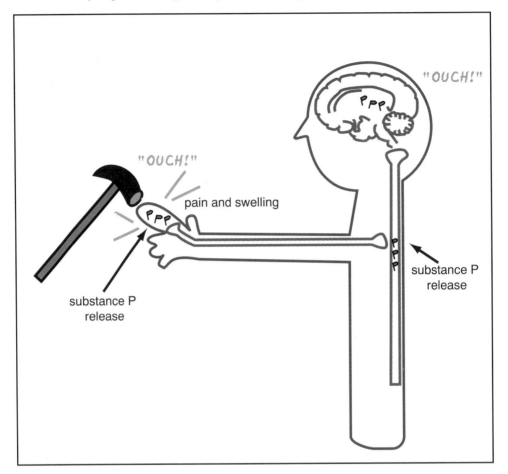

FIGURE 1–65. Classically, **substance P** was thought to be involved in the **pain** response because it is released from neurons in peripheral tissues in response to inflammation, causing "neurogenic" inflammation and pain. Furthermore, substance P is present in spinal pain pathways, which suggests a role in central nervous system–medicated pain. Unfortunately, however, antagonists to substance P's receptors were unable to reduce neurogenic inflammation or pain of many types in human testing.

drugs might be effective in reducing emotional distress has nevertheless spawned a race to find antagonists for all three of the known neurokinins to see if they would have therapeutic actions in a wide variety of psychiatric disorders. Substance P and its related neurokinins are present in areas of the brain such as the amygdala that are thought to be critical for regulating emotions (Fig. 1–66). The neurokinins are also present in areas of the brain rich with monoamines, which suggests a potential regulatory role of neurokinins for monoamine neurotransmitters already known to be important in numerous psychiatric disorders and in the mechanisms of action of numerous psychotropic drugs. Thus, antagonists to all three important neurokinins are currently in clinical testing of various states of emotional dysfunction, including depression, anxiety, and schizophrenia. Over the next few years it should become apparent whether this strategy can be exploited to generate truly novel psychotropic drugs acting on an entirely new neurotransmitter system, namely, the neurokinins.

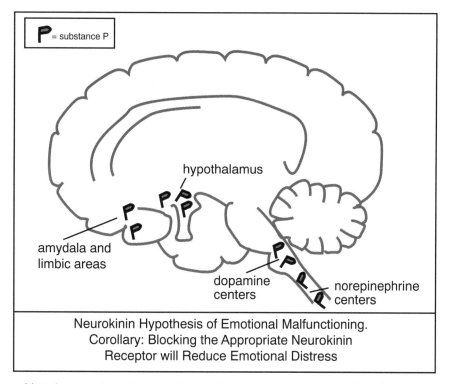

Neurokinin Hypothesis of Emotional Malfunctioning.
Corollary: Blocking the Appropriate Neurokinin
Receptor will Reduce Emotional Distress

FIGURE 1–66. **Substance P** and its related neurokinins are present in areas of the brain such as the amygdala that are thought to be critical for regulating **emotions**. The neurokinins are also present in areas of the brain rich in monoamines, which suggests a potential regulatory role of monoamine neurotransmitters, which are already known to be important in numerous psychiatric disorders and in the mechanisms of action of numerous psychotropic drugs.

Substance P and neurokinin 1 receptors. The first neurokinin was discovered in the 1930s in extracts of brain or intestine. Since it was prepared as a "powder," it was called substance P. This molecule is now known to be a string of 11 amino acids (an undecapeptide) (Fig. 1–67). This is in sharp contrast to monoamine neurotransmitters, which are modifications of a single amino acid.

The following are some of the differences between the synthesis of neurotransmitter by a monoaminergic neuron and by a peptidergic neuron. Whereas monoamines are made from dietary amino acids, peptide neurotransmitters are made from proteins that are direct gene products. However, genes are not translated directly into peptide neurotransmitters but into precursors of the peptide neurotransmitters. These precursors are sometimes called "grandparent" proteins, or pre-propeptides. Further modifications convert these grandparent proteins into the direct precursors of peptide neurotransmitters, sometimes called the "parents" of the neuropeptide, or the propeptides. Finally, modifications of the parental peptide produces the neuropeptide progeny itself.

For neurons utilizing substance P, synthesis starts with the gene called pre-protachykinin A (PPT-A) (Fig. 1–68). This gene is transcribed into RNA, which is then "edited," or revised by cutting and pasting, like revising a manuscript or a

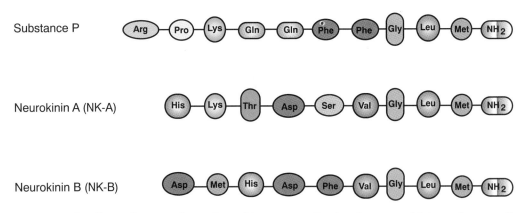

FIGURE 1–67. Shown here are the amino acid sequences for the three neurokinins **substance P**, **neurokinin A** (NK-A) and **neurokinin B** (NK-B). Substance P has 11 amino acid units and NK-A and NK-B each have 10. Several of the amino acids are the same in these three peptides.

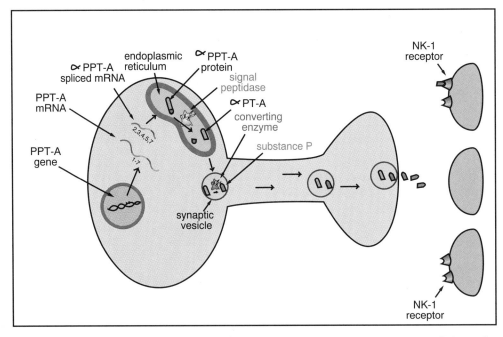

FIGURE 1–68. Substance P neurons and neurokinin 1 receptors, part 1. For neurons utilizing **substance P**, synthesis starts with the gene called pre-protachykinin A (**PPT-A**). This gene is transcribed into RNA, which is then "edited" to form three alternative mRNA splice variants, alpha, beta, and gamma. The actions of the mRNA version called alpha-PPT-A mRNA are shown here. This mRNA is then transcribed into a protein called alpha-PPT-A, which is substance P's "grandparent." It is converted in the endoplasmic reticulum into the "parent" of substance P, called protachykinin A (alpha-PT-A). Finally, this protein is clipped even shorter by another enzyme, called a converting enzyme, in the synaptic vesicle and forms substance P itself.

videotape. Thus, this process is sometimes called "splicing" of the RNA. This leads to different versions of RNA called *alternative mRNA splice variants*.

The mRNA version called alpha-PPT-A mRNA goes on to be transcribed into a protein called alpha-PPT-A, which is substance P's grandparent (Fig. 1–68). It is much longer than substance P itself, as it contains a longer string of amino acids. The alpha-PPT-A grandparent protein needs to be cut down to size by an enzyme in the endoplasmic reticulum called a *signal peptidase*. Thus, pro-tachykinin A (alpha-PT-A) protein is formed, the parent of substance P. Finally, alpha PT-A is clipped even shorter by another enzyme in the synaptic vesicle called a *converting enzyme*, and forms substance P itself (Fig. 1–68).

Substance P can also be formed from two other proteins, called beta-PPT-A and gamma PPT-A (Figs. 1–69 and 1–70). These proteins come from different mRNA splice variants, but the same precursor PPT-A gene. Not only can substance P be formed from these proteins, but so can another important neurokinin, called neurokinin A (NK-A) (Figs. 1–71 and 1–72). Thus, substance P can be formed from three proteins derived from the PPT-A gene, namely, alpha, beta, and gamma PPT-A (Figs. 1–68 to 1–70), and NK-A can be formed from two of these, beta and gamma PPT-A (Figs. 1–71 and 1–72).

Substance P is released from neurons and prefers to interact selectively with the neurokinin 1 (NK-1) subtype of neurokinin receptor (Figs. 1–68 to 1–70). Inter-

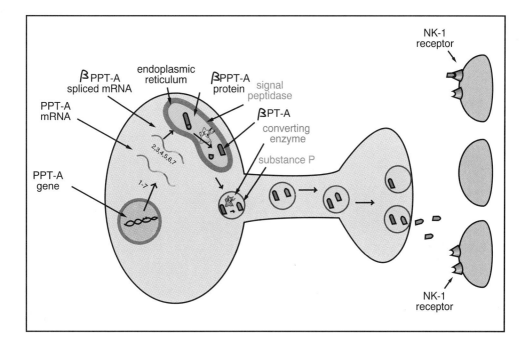

FIGURE 1–69. Substance P and neurokinin 1 receptors, part 2. **Substance P** can also be formed from two other proteins, called **beta-PPT-A**, shown here, and gamma PPT-A, shown in Figure 1–70. These proteins come from different mRNA splice variants but the same precursor PPT-A gene.

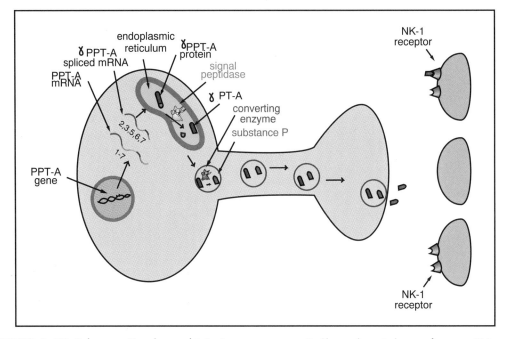

FIGURE 1−70. Substance P and neurokinin 1 receptors, part 3. Shown here is how **substance P** is formed from **gamma PPT-A**. Thus, substance P can be formed from three proteins derived from the PPT-A gene, namely, alpha, beta, and gamma PPT-A (see also Figs. 1−68 and 1−69). When substance P is released from neurons, it prefers to interact selectively with the **neurokinin** 1 subtype of neurokinin receptor (Figs. 1−68 to 1−70). However, there is a mismatch in the brain between the locations of substance P and the NK-1 receptors, suggesting that substance P acts preferentially by volume neurotransmission at sites remote from its axon terminals rather than by classical synaptic neurotransmission.

estingly, however, there is a bit of a mismatch in the brain between where substance P is located and where the NK-1 receptors are located. This may suggest that substance P acts preferentially by volume neurotransmission at sites remote from its axon terminals rather than by classical synaptic neurotransmission.

Neurokinin A and neurokinin 2 receptors. Neurokinin A (NK-A) is another member of the neurokinin family of peptide neurotransmitters. It is a peptide containing 10 amino acid units (decapeptide), with 5 amino acid units the same as in substance P, including 4 of the last 5 on its N-terminal tail (Fig. 1−67). As mentioned above, it is formed both from the beta and the gamma PPT-A proteins derived from the PPT-A gene (Figs. 1−71 and 1−72). The beta and gamma PPT-A proteins are the grandparents of NK-A and are cut down to size just as described for substance P, eventually forming the peptide neurotransmitter NK-A.

This neurokinin prefers a different receptor than does substance P. Thus, NK-A specifically binds the NK-2 receptor (Figs. 1−71 and 1−72). There are few NK-A receptors in the brain of rats, so the guinea pig is a closer model to humans, with

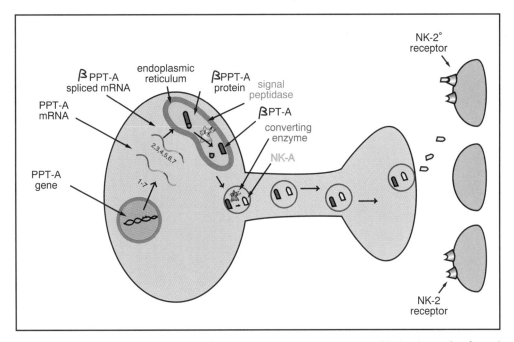

FIGURE 1–71. Neurokinin A and neurokinin 2 receptors, part 1. **Neurokinin A** can be formed from two of the same proteins that form substance P, namely beta and gamma PPT-A. The formation of neurokinin A from **beta PPT-A** is shown here.

NK-A receptors also in peripheral tissues such as the lung. As for substance P, there is a mismatch between the neurotransmitter and its receptor anatomically, which suggests the important role of nonsynaptic volume neurotransmission for NK-A as well. However, the anatomical distribution of NK-A is different from that of substance P, and the anatomical distribution of NK-2 receptors is different from that of NK-1 receptors.

Neurokinin B and neurokinin B receptors. The third important member of the neurokinin neurotransmitter family is neurokinin B (NK-B). Like NK-A, it is a ten amino acid peptide (decapeptide). Six of the ten amino acids in NK-B are the same as in NK-A, and four of the last five amino acids in the N-terminal tail of NK-B are identical to substance P (Fig. 1–67).

Neurokinin B is formed from a gene called PPT-B, which is different from that from which substance P and NK-A are derived. However, the process of converting the PPT-B protein into NK-B is analogous to that already described for substance P and NK-A (Fig. 1–73). NK-B prefers its own unique receptors, called NK-3 receptors (Fig. 1–73). Neurokinin B and its NK-3 receptors are also mismatched, and in different anatomical areas from substance P, NK-A, and their NK-1 and NK-2 receptors, respectively.

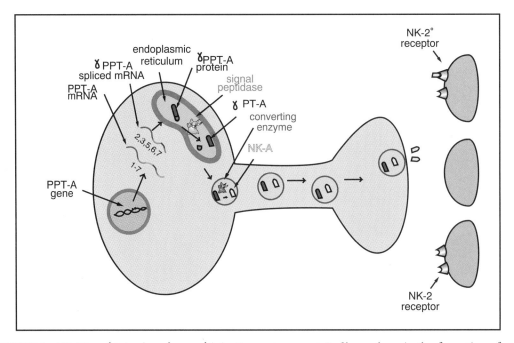

FIGURE 1–72. Neurokinin A and neurokinin 2 receptors, part 2. Shown here is the formation of **NK-A from the gamma PPT-A protein**. The beta and gamma PPT-A proteins are the "grandparents" of NK-A and are cut down to size just as described for substance P, eventually forming the peptide neurotransmitter NK-A. Neurokinin A specifically binds to the **NK-2 receptor**. As for substance P, there is a mismatch between this neurotransmitter and its receptor anatomically, suggesting the important role of nonsynaptic volume neurotransmission for NK-A as well. However, the anatomical distribution of NK-A is different from that of substance P, and the anatomical distribution of NK-2 receptors is different from that of NK-1 receptors.

Summary

In this chapter we have introduced two major psychopharmacological themes, namely, the affective disorders and the monoamine and neuropeptide neurotransmitters. We have described the clinical features, epidemiology, and longitudinal course of various types of depression, including the impact that treatments are having on the long-term outcome of affective disorders. We have also described the three monoamine neurotransmitter systems—noradrenergic, dopaminergic, and serotonergic. Specifically, the synthesis, metabolism, transport systems, and receptors for each monoaminergic system have been outlined and then applied to the leading theories for the biological basis of depression. These theories of depression are the monoamine hypothesis, the neurotransmitter hypothesis, and the pseudomonoamine hypothesis of defective signal transduction and gene expression. Finally, we have introduced a new family of neurotransmitters and their receptors, called neurokinins, of which substance P is the most prominent member.

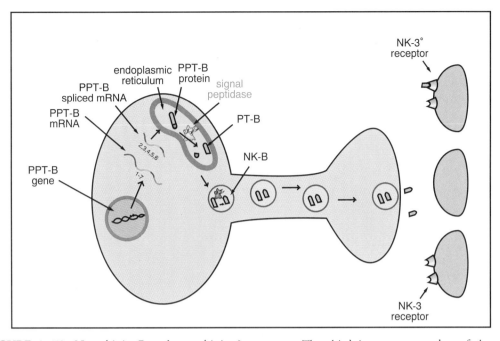

FIGURE 1–73. Neurokinin B and neurokinin 3 receptors. The third important member of the neurokinin neurotransmitter family is **NK-B**, which is formed from a gene, called **PPT-B**, which is different from the gene from which either substance P or NK-A is derived. However, the process of converting the PPT-B protein into NK-B is analogous to that already described for substance P and NK-A. Neurokinin B prefers its own unique receptors, called **NK-3 receptors**. Neurokinin B and its NK-3 receptors are also mismatched and are located in different anatomical areas from substance P, NK-A, and their NK-1 and NK-2 receptors, respectively.

The material in this chapter should provide the reader with the basis for under-standing the pharmacologic basis of the treatment of depression discussed in the following two chapters. It should also provide useful background information about the monoamine neurotransmitter systems that serve as the pharmacological basis for several other classes of psychotropic drugs.

CHAPTER 2

CLASSICAL ANTIDEPRESSANTS, SEROTONIN SELECTIVE REUPTAKE INHIBITORS, AND NORADRENERGIC REUPTAKE INHIBITORS

In this chapter, we will review pharmacological concepts underlying the use of several classes of antidepressant drugs, including the classical monoamine oxidase (MAO) inhibitors, the classical tricyclic antidepressants, the popular serotonin selective reuptake inhibitors (SSRIs), and the new selective noradrenergic reuptake inhibitors, as well as norepinephrine and dopamine reuptake inhibitors. The goal of this chapter is to acquaint the reader with current ideas about how these antidepressants work. We will explain the mechanisms of action of these drugs by building on general pharmacological concepts. We will also introduce pharmacokinetic concepts for the antidepressants, namely, how the body acts on these drugs through the cytochrome P450 enzyme system.

Our treatment of antidepressants in this chapter is at the conceptual level and not at the pragmatic level. The reader should consult standard drug handbooks for details of doses, side effects, drug interactions, and other issues relevant to the prescribing of these drugs in clinical practice.

Theories of Antidepressant Drug Action

Classifications Based on Acute Pharmacological Actions

We do not currently have a complete and adequate explanation of how antidepressant drugs work. What we do know is that all effective antidepressants have identifiable immediate interactions with one or more monoamine neurotransmitter receptor or enzyme. These immediate actions provide the pharmacological foundation for the current classification of the different antidepressants.

According to this classification scheme, there are at least eight separate pharmacological mechanisms of action and more than two dozen antidepressants. Most antidepressants block monoamine reuptake, but some block alpha 2 receptors and others the enzyme monoamine oxidase (MAO). Some antidepressants have direct actions on only one monoamine neurotransmitter system; others have direct actions on more than one monoamine neurotransmitter system. As discussed in Chapter 1, the immediate pharmacological actions of all antidepressants eventually have the effect of boosting the levels of monoamine neurotransmitters (Figs. 1–15 and 1–16; see also Fig. 2–1). This chapter and the following chapter will review those specific receptors and enzymes that are influenced by each of the various antidepressants immediately after administration to a depressed patient. Just how all these different immediate pharmacological actions result ultimately in an antidepressant response a few weeks after administration of an antidepressant agent—that is, the final common pathway of antidepressant treatment response—is the subject of intense research interest and debate (Fig. 2–1). Currently, there is intense focus on the gene expression that is triggered by antidepressants. The monoamine hypothesis of antidepressant action on gene expression suggests that gene expression is ultimately the most important action of antidepressants.

The Neurotransmitter Receptor Hypothesis of Antidepressant Action

One theory to explain the ultimate mechanism of delayed therapeutic action of antidepressants is the neurotransmitter receptor hypothesis of antidepressant action (Figs. 2–1 through 2–6). This is a hypothesis related to the neurotransmitter receptor hypothesis of depression discussed in Chapter 1 (Figs. 1–60 through 1–62). As previously discussed, this latter hypothesis proposes that depression itself is linked to abnormal functioning of neurotransmitter receptors.

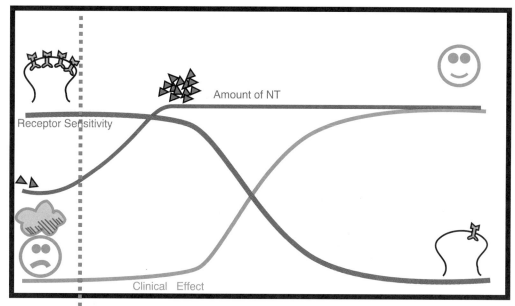

Antidepressant introduced

FIGURE 2–1. This figure depicts the different time courses for three effects of antidepressant drugs, namely clinical changes, neurotransmitter (NT) changes, and receptor sensitivity changes. Specifically, the **amount of NT** changes relatively rapidly after an **antidepressant is introduced**. However, the **clinical effect** is delayed, as is the desensitization, or down regulation, of neurotransmitter **receptors**. This temporal correlation of clinical effects with changes in receptor sensitivity has given rise to the hypothesis that changes in neurotransmitter receptor sensitivity may actually mediate the clinical effects of antidepressant drugs. These clinical effects include not only antidepressant and anxiolytic actions but also the development of tolerance to the acute side effects of antidepressant drugs.

    Whether or not neurotransmitter receptors are abnormal in depression, the neurotransmitter receptor hypothesis of antidepressant action proposes that antidepressants, no matter what their initial actions on receptors and enzymes, eventually cause a desensitization, or down regulation, of key neurotransmitter receptors in a time course consistent with the delayed onset of antidepressant action of these drugs (Figs. 2–1 through 2–6).

    This time course coincides with other events, including the time it takes for a patient to become tolerant to the side effects of antidepressants. Thus, desensitization of some neurotransmitter receptors may lead to the delayed therapeutic actions of antidepressants, whereas desensitization of other neurotransmitter receptors may lead to the decrease of side effects over time.

    An overly simplistic view of the neurotransmitter receptor hypothesis of depression is that the normal state becomes one of depression as neurotransmitter is depleted and postsynaptic receptors then up-regulate (Fig. 2–2). Boosting neurotransmitters by MAO inhibition (Figs. 2–3 and 2–4) or by blocking reuptake pumps for monoamine neurotransmitters (Figs. 2–5 and 2–6) eventually results in the down regulation of neurotransmitter receptors in a delayed time course more closely related to the timing of recovery from depression (Figs. 2–1, 2–4, and 2–6).

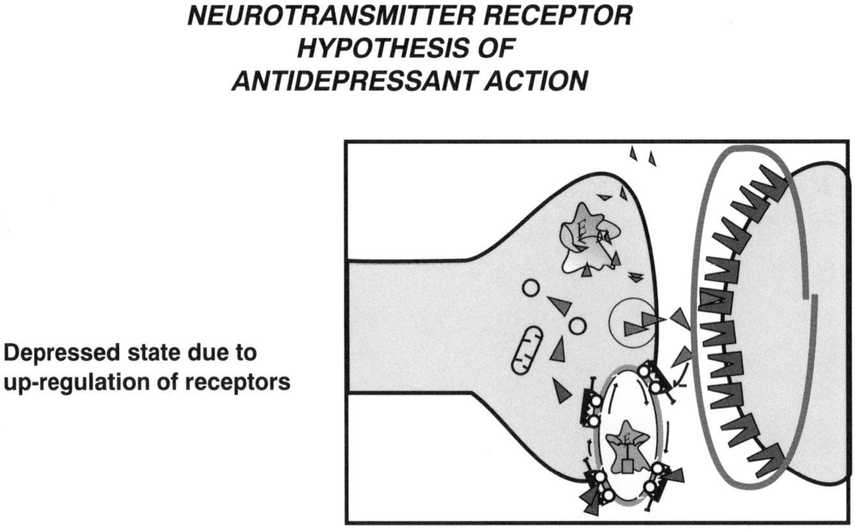

NEUROTRANSMITTER RECEPTOR
HYPOTHESIS OF
ANTIDEPRESSANT ACTION

**Depressed state due to
up-regulation of receptors**

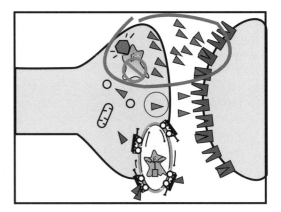

FIGURE 2–2. *The neurotransmitter receptor hypothesis of antidepressant action*—**part 1.** Shown here is the monoaminergic neuron in the **depressed state**, with **up regulation of receptors** (indicated in the red circle).

NEUROTRANSMITTER RECEPTOR
HYPOTHESIS OF
ANTIDEPRESSANT ACTION

**MAO Inhibitor
tells the enzyme
to stop destroying NE**

FIGURE 2–3. *The neurotransmitter receptor hypothesis of antidepressant action*—**part 2.** Here, a monoamine oxidase (**MAO**) **inhibitor** is blocking the enzyme and thereby stopping the destruction of neurotransmitter. This causes **more neurotransmitter to be available** in the synapse (indicated in the red circle).

Originally, it was hypothesized that desensitization of postsynaptic receptors may be responsible for the therapeutic actions of antidepressants. It is now clear that desensitization of some postsynaptic receptors is responsible for the development of tolerance to the acute side effects of antidepressants. Attention is currently being

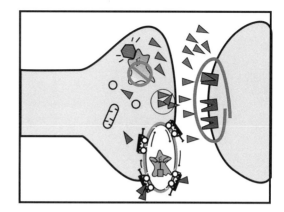

Increase in NT causes receptors to down-regulate

FIGURE 2–4. *The neurotransmitter receptor hypothesis of antidepressant action*—part 3. The consequence of **long-lasting blockade** of monoamine oxidase (**MAO**) by an MAO inhibitor is that the neurotransmitter **receptors are desensitized or down-regulated** (indicated in the red circle).

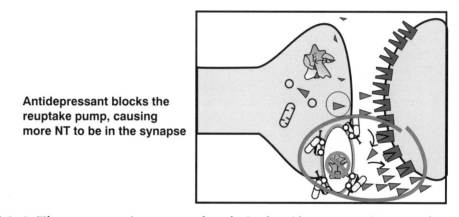

Antidepressant blocks the reuptake pump, causing more NT to be in the synapse

FIGURE 2–5. *The neurotransmitter receptor hypothesis of antidepressant action*—part 4. Here, a **tricyclic antidepressant** blocks the reuptake pump, causing **more neurotransmitter** to be available in the synapse (indicated in the red circle). This is very similar to what happens after MAO is inhibited (Fig. 2–3).

focused on the presynaptic receptors and their desensitization in order to explain the therapeutic actions of antidepressants. This will be discussed in more detail in the section on serotonin selective reuptake inhibitors (SSRIs).

The Monoamine Hypothesis of Antidepressant Action on Gene Expression

As discussed in Chapter 1 (Figs. 1–63 and 1–64), the monoamine hypothesis of gene expression proposes that depression itself is linked to abnormal functioning of neurotransmitter-inducible gene expression, particularly neurotrophic factors such as

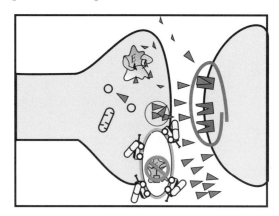

Increase in NT causes receptors to down-regulate

FIGURE 2–6. *The neurotransmitter receptor hypothesis of antidepressant action*—part 5. The consequence of **long-lasting blockade** of the reuptake pump by a **tricyclic antidepressant** is to cause the neurotransmitter **receptors to become desensitized or down-regulated** (indicated in the red circle). This is the same outcome as with long-lasting blockade of MAO (see Fig. 2–4).

brain-derived neurotrophic factor (BDNF), leading to atrophy and apoptosis of critical hippocampal neurons. Whether or not the transduction of a monoaminergic neuronal impulse into gene expression is actually abnormal in depression, the monoamine hypothesis of antidepressant action on gene expression proposes that antidepressants, no matter what their initial actions on receptors and enzymes, eventually cause critical genes to be activated or inactivated. One of these may indeed be BDNF, although many others are undoubtedly involved as well (Fig. 2–7). Changes in the genetic expression of monoamine neurotransmitter receptors have already been discussed (Figs. 2–1 through 2–6). Thus, the gene expression hypothesis is consistent with the monoamine receptor hypothesis of antidepressant action but is broader in scope.

Delayed actions of antidepressants may not only explain the delay in onset of therapeutic action of antidepressants; they may also explain why some patients fail to respond to antidepressants, since it is possible that in such patients the initial pharmacological actions are not translated into the required delayed pharmacologic and genetic actions. Knowing the biological basis for treatment nonresponse may lead to a greatly needed advance in the pharmacotherapy of depression, namely an effective treatment for refractory or nonresponding depressed patients, as discussed in Chapter 1. Also, if one understands the key pharmacologic events that are linked to the therapeutic actions of the drugs, it may be possible to accelerate them with future drugs. If so, it could lead to another highly desired advance in the pharmacotherapy of depression, namely a rapid-onset antidepressant.

In summary, all antidepressants have a common action on monoamine neurotransmitters—they boost monoamine neurotransmission, leading to changes in gene expression in the neurons targeted by the monoamines. This includes desensitization of neurotransmitter receptors, leading to both therapeutic action and tolerance to side effects. Although antidepressants are classified on the basis of those actions on neurotransmitter receptors and enzymes that are immediate, attention is increasingly being paid to how these initial and immediate actions translate into delayed actions.

Monoamine Hypothesis of Antidepresssant Action on Gene Expression

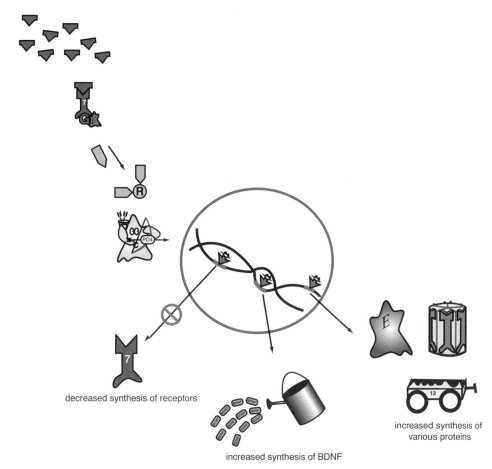

decreased synthesis of receptors

increased synthesis of BDNF

increased synthesis of various proteins

FIGURE 2–7. The **monoamine hypothesis of antidepressant action on gene expression** is shown here. The neurotransmitter at the top is presumably increased by an antidepressant. The cascading consequence of this is ultimately to change the expression of critical genes in order to effect an antidepressant response. This includes down-regulating some genes so that there is decreased synthesis of receptors, as well as up-regulating other genes so that there is increased synthesis of critical proteins, such as brain-derived neurotrophic factor (BDNF).

Pharmacokinetics of Antidepressants

Recently, there has been a rapid increase in our knowledge about how antidepressants and mood stabilizers are metabolized and about drug interactions with antidepressants and mood stabilizers. *Pharmacokinetics* is the study of how the body acts on drugs, especially to absorb, distribute, metabolize, and excrete them. These pharmacokinetic actions are mediated through the hepatic and gut drug-metabolizing system known as the cytochrome P450 (CYP450) enzyme system.

The CYP450 enzymes and the *pharmacokinetic* actions they represent must be contrasted with the *pharmacodynamic* actions of antidepressants, which were discussed in the previous section on the mechanism of action of antidepressants. Although

Table 2–1. *Pharmacokinetics and pharmacodynamics*

PHARMACOKINETICS:
How the body acts on drugs
PHARMACODYNAMICS:
How drugs act on the body, especially the brain

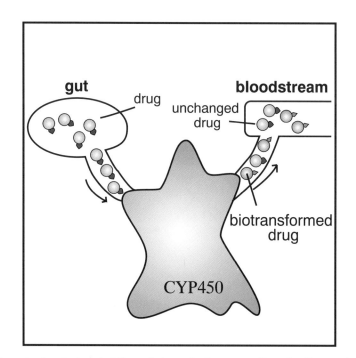

FIGURE 2–8. A **drug** is absorbed and delivered through the gut wall to the liver to be **biotransformed** so that it can be excreted. Specifically, the **cytochrome P450 (CYP450)** enzyme in the gut wall or liver converts the drug substrate into a biotransformed product in the bloodstream. After passing through the gut wall and liver (left), the drug will exist partly as unchanged drug and partly as biotransformed drug (right).

most of this book deals with the *pharmacodynamics* of psychopharmacological agents, especially how these drugs act on the brain, the following section will discuss the *pharmacokinetics* of antidepressants and mood stabilizers, or how the body acts on these drugs (Table 2–1).

The CYP450 enzymes follow the principle of transforming substrates into products. Figure 2–8 shows how an antidepressant is absorbed and delivered through the gut wall to the liver to be biotransformed so that it can be excreted from the body. Specifically, the CYP450 enzyme in the gut wall or liver converts the drug substrate into a biotransformed product in the bloodstream. After passing through the gut wall and liver, the drug will exist partly as unchanged drug and partly as biotransformed product (Fig. 2–8).

There are several known CYP450 systems. Five of the most important enzymes for antidepressant drug metabolism are shown in Figure 2–9. There are over 30

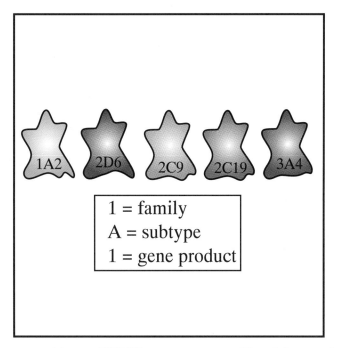

FIGURE 2–9. There are several known **CYP450 enzyme systems**. Five of the most important for antidepressant and mood stabilizer metabolism are shown here.

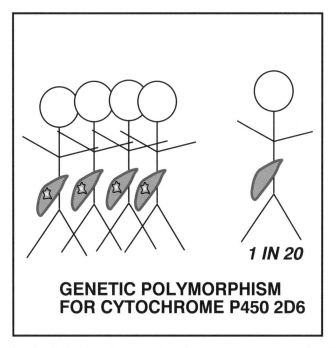

FIGURE 2–10. Not all individuals have the same CYP450 enzymes. For example, about 1 in 20 Caucausians is a **poor metabolizer via 2D6** and must metabolize drugs by an alternative route, which may not be as efficient.

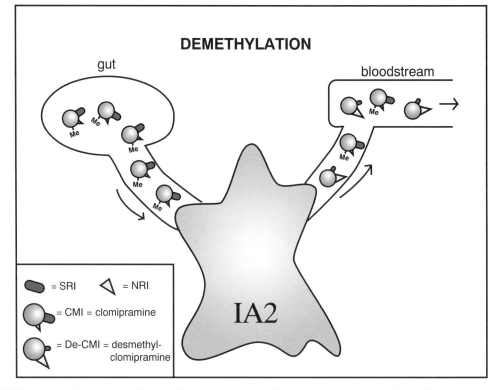

FIGURE 2–11. Certain tricyclic antidepressants, especially secondary amines such as clomipramine and imipramine, are substrates for **CYP450 1A2**. This enzyme converts the tricyclics into active metabolites by demethylation to form desmethylclomipramine and desipramine, respectively.

known CYP450 enzymes, and probably many more awaiting discovery and classification. Not all individuals have all the same CYP450 enzymes. In such cases, the enzyme is said to be polymorphic. For example, about 5 to 10% of Caucasians are poor metabolizers via the enzyme CYP450 2D6 (Fig. 2–10). They must metabolize drugs by alternative routes, which may not be as efficient as the CYP450 2D6 route. Another CYP450 enzyme, 2C19, has reduced activity in approximately 20% of Japanese and Chinese individuals and in 3 to 5% of Caucasians.

CYP450 1A2

One CYP450 enzyme of relevance to antidepressants is 1A2 (Figs. 2–11 and 2–12). Certain tricyclic antidepressants (TCAs) are *substrates* for this enzyme, especially the secondary amines such as clomipramine and imipramine (Fig. 2–11). CYP450 1A2 demethylates such TCAs, but does not thereby inactivate them. In these cases, the desmethyl metabolite of the TCA (e.g., desmethylclomipramine and desipramine) is still an active drug (Fig. 2–12).

CYP450 1A2 is *inhibited* by the serotonin selective reuptake inhibitor fluvoxamine (Fig. 2–12) Thus, when fluvoxamine is given concomitantly with other drugs that use 1A2 for their metabolism, those drugs can no longer be metabolized as efficiently.

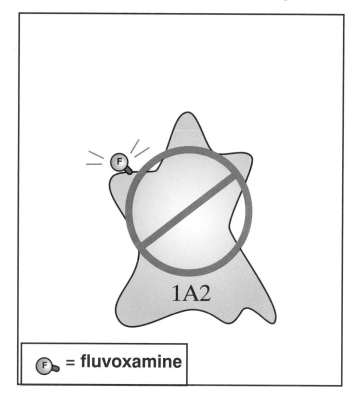

FIGURE 2–12. The SSRI **fluvoxamine** is a potent **inhibitor** of the enzyme CYP450 1A2.

An example of a potentially important drug interaction is that which occurs when fluvoxamine is given along with theophyllin (Figure 2–13). In that case, the theophyllin dose must be lowered or else the blood levels of theophyllin will rise and possibly cause side effects, even toxic side effects such as seizures. The same may occur with caffeine. Fluvoxamine also affects the metabolism of atypical antipsychotics.

CYP450 2D6

Another important CYP450 enzyme for antidepressants is 2D6. Tricyclic antidepressants are *substrates* for 2D6, which hydroxylates and thereby inactivates them (Fig. 2–14). Several antidepressants from the SSRI class are *inhibitors* of CYP2D6 (Fig. 2–15). There is a wide range of potency for 2D6 inhibition by the five SSRIs, with paroxetine and fluoxetine the most potent and fluvoxamine, sertraline, and citalopram the least potent.

One of the most important drug interactions that SSRIs can cause through inhibition of 2D6 is to raise plasma levels of tricyclic antidepressants (TCAs) if these TCAs are given concomitantly with SSRIs or if there is switching between TCAs and SSRIs. Since TCAs are substrates for 2D6 (Fig. 2–14) and SSRIs are inhibitors of 2D6 (Fig. 2–15), concomitant administration will raise TCA levels, perhaps to toxic levels (Fig. 2–16). Concomitant administration of an SSRI and a TCA thus

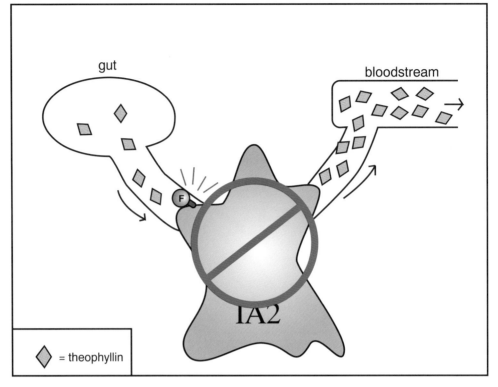

FIGURE 2–13. **Theophyllin** is a **substrate** for CYP450 1A2. Thus, in the presence of the 1A2 inhibitor **fluvoxamine**, theophyllin levels rise. The theophyllin dose must be lowered when it is given with fluvoxamine in order to avoid side effects.

requires monitoring of the plasma drug concentrations of the TCA and probably a reduction in its dose. CYP450 2D6 also interacts with atypical antipsychotics.

CYP450 3A4

A third important CYP450 enzyme for antidepressants and mood stabilizers is 3A4. Some benzodiazepines (e.g., alprazolam and triazolam) are *substrates* for 3A4 (Fig. 2–17). Some antidepressants are 3A4 *inhibitors*, including the SSRIs fluoxetine and fluvoxamine and the antidepressant nefazodone (Fig. 2–18). Administration of a 3A4 substrate with a 3A4 inhibitor will raise the level of the substrate. For example, fluoxetine, fluvoxamine, or nefazodone will raise the levels of alprazolam or triazolam, requiring dose reduction of the benzodiazepine (Fig. 2–18).

Other nonpsychotropic drugs are also substrates (Fig. 2–17) or inhibitors of 3A4 (Fig. 2–18). It is important to understand the consequences of concomitant administration of psychotropic drugs that are either substrates or inhibitors of 3A4 with nonpsychotropic drugs that are also either substrates or inhibitors of 3A4. Notably, some 3A4 substrates such as cisapride, terfenidine, and astemazole must be metabolized, or else toxic levels of the drug can accumulate, with cardiovascular consequences such as prolonged QT interval and sudden death. Thus, they cannot be

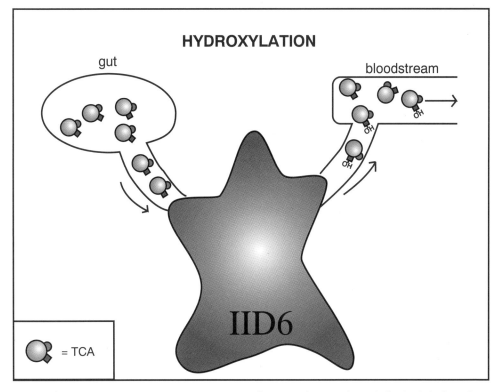

HYDROXYLATION

gut

bloodstream

IID6

= TCA

FIGURE 2–14. Tricyclic antidepressants (TCAs) are **substrates** for CYP450 **2D6**, which hydroxylates and thereby inactivates them.

given with a 3A4 inhibitor because of this potential danger, and use of fluoxetine, fluvoxamine, and nefazodone with such 3A4 substrates must be avoided. Changes in 3A4 activity also affect atypical antipsychotic drug levels.

CYP450 Inducers

Finally, not only can drugs be substrates or inhibitors for CYP450 enzymes; they can also be *inducers*. An inducer increases the activity of the enzyme over time because it induces the synthesis of more copies of the enzyme. One example of this is the effects of the anticonvulsant and mood stabilizer carbamazepine, which induces 3A4 over time (Fig. 2–19). Another example of CYP450 enzyme induction is cigarette smoking, which induces 1A2 over time (Fig. 2–20). The consequence of such enzyme induction is that substrates for the induced enzyme will be more efficiently metabolized over time, and thus their levels in the plasma will fall. Doses of such substrate drugs may therefore need to be increased over time to compensate for this.

For example carbamazepine is both a substrate and an inducer of 3A4. Thus as treatment becomes chronic, 3A4 is induced and carbamazepine blood levels fall (Fig. 2–19). Failure to recognize this effect and to increase carbamazepine dosage to compensate for it may lead to a failure of anticonvulsant or mood-stabilizing efficacy, with breakthrough symptoms.

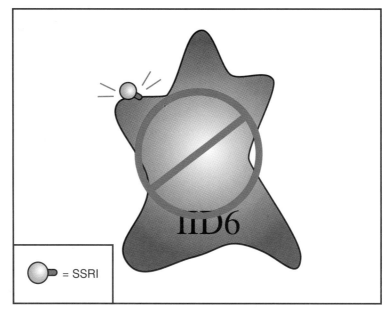

FIGURE 2–15. Some serotonin selective reuptake inhibitors (SSRIs) are **inhibitors** of CYP450 **2D6**. Fluoxetine and paroxetine are potent **inhibitors** of 2D6, and fluvoxamine, sertaline, and citalopram are weak inhibitors of 2D6.

Another important thing to remember about a CYP450 inducer is what happens if the inducer is stopped. Thus, if one stops smoking, 1A2 substrate levels will rise. If one stops carbamazepine, the plasma concentrations will rise for any concomitantly administered drug that is a 3A4 substrate.

An overview of some actions of antidepressants at various CYP450 enzyme systems is given in Table 2–2. This is not a comprehensive list, and the discussion here has only been at the conceptual level, leaving out many important details that the prescriber will need to know. In this rapidly evolving area of therapeutics, the only way to keep up is to continually consult updated standard reference materials on drug interactions and the specific dosing implications that such interactions cause. In summary (Table 2–3), many drug interactions require dosage adjustment of one of the drugs. A few combinations must be strictly avoided. Many drug interactions are statistically significant but not clinically significant. By following the principles outlined here, the skilled practitioner and antidepressant prescriber must learn whether any given drug interaction is clinically relevant.

Classical Antidepressants: Monoamine Oxidase Inhibitors and Tricyclic Antidepressants

Monoamine Oxidase Inhibitors

The first clinically effective antidepressants to be discovered were immediate inhibitors of the enzyme monoamine oxidase (MAO) (Table 2–4 and Figs. 1–15, 2–3, and 2–4). They were discovered by accident when an antituberculosis drug was

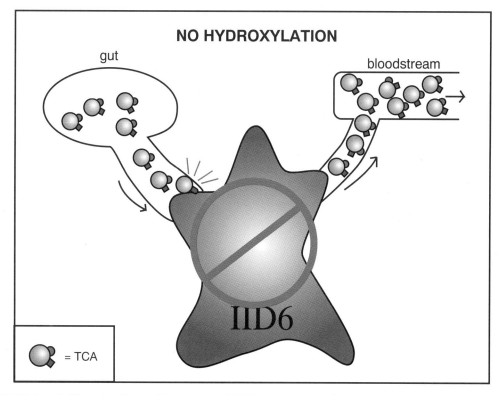

NO HYDROXYLATION

gut

bloodstream

IID6

= TCA

FIGURE 2–16. If a **tricyclic antidepressant** (TCA) is given together with a **serotonin selective reuptake inhibitor** (SSRI), the SSRI will prevent TCA metabolism. This causes TCA levels to increase, which can be toxic. Therefore either monitoring of TCA plasma concentration with dose reduction of the TCA, or avoidance of the combination, is required.

observed to help depression that coexisted in some of the tuberculosis patients. This antituberculosis drug, which was also an antidepressant, was soon discovered to inhibit the enzyme MAO. It was soon thereafter shown that inhibition of MAO was unrelated to its antitubercular actions but was the immediate biochemical event that caused its ultimate antidepressant actions. This discovery soon led to the synthesis of more drugs in the 1950s and 1960s that inhibited MAO but lacked unwanted additional properties, such as antituberculosis properties. Although best known as powerful antidepressants, the MAO inhibitors are also therapeutic agents for certain anxiety disorders, such as panic disorder and social phobia.

The original MAO inhibitors are all irreversible enzyme inhibitors, which bind to MAO irreversibly and destroy its function forever. Enzyme activity returns only after new enzyme is synthesized (see Figs. 1–15, 2–3 and 2–4). Sometimes such inhibitors are called "suicide inhibitors" because once the enzyme binds the inhibitor, the enzyme essentially commits suicide in that it can never function again until a new enzyme protein is synthesized by the neuron's DNA in the cell nucleus.

Monoamine oxidase exists in two subtypes, A and B. Both forms are inhibited by the original MAO inhibitors, which are therefore nonselective. The A form metabolizes the neurotransmitter monoamines most closely linked to depression (serotonin and norepinephrine).

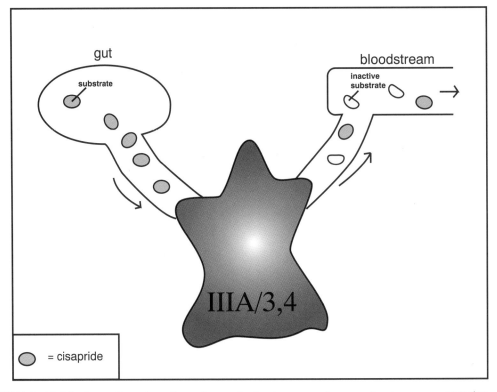

FIGURE 2–17. The benzodiazepines alprazolam and triazolam are **substrates** for the enzyme CYP450 3A4. The nonpsychotropic drugs cisapride and astemazole are also substrates for 3A4.

It thereby also metabolizes the amine most closely linked to control of blood pressure (norepinephrine). The B form is thought to convert some amine substrates, called protoxins, into toxins that may cause damage to neurons. Because of these observations, MAO A inhibition is linked both to antidepressant action and to the troublesome hypertensive side effects of the MAO inhibitors. Inhibition of MAO B is linked to prevention of neurodegenerative processes, such as those in Parkinson's disease.

Two developments have occurred with MAO inhibitors in recent years. One is the production of selective inhibitors of MAO A or of MAO B. The other advance is the production of selective MAO A inhibitors that are reversible. The implications of these advances are multiple. One of the most troublesome properties of the original nonselective, irreversible MAO inhibitors is the fact that after they inhibit MAO, amines taken in from the diet can cause dangerous elevations in blood pressure. Normally, such dietary amines are safely metabolized by MAO before they can cause blood pressure elevations (Figs. 2–21 and 2–22). However, when MAO A is inhibited, blood pressure can rise suddenly and dramatically and can even cause intracerebral hemorrhage and death after consumption of certain tyramine-containing foods or beverages (Fig. 2–23). This risk can be controlled by restricting the diet so that dangerous foods are eliminated and also restricting the simultaneous dangerous use of certain medications (e.g., the pain killer meperidine [Demerol]; the

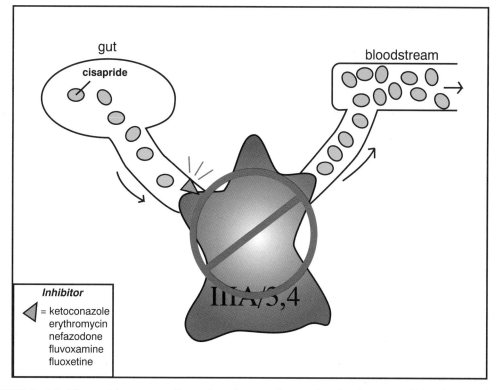

FIGURE 2–18. The antidepressants fluoxetine, fluvoxamine, and nefazodone are all **inhibitors** of CYP450 3A4. More potent inhibitors of this enzyme include the nonpsychotropic drugs ketoconazole, erythromycin, and protease inhibitors. If a 3A4 inhibitor is given with cisapride or astemazole, levels of these substrates can rise to toxic levels. Thus, fluoxetine, fluvoxamine, and nefazodone cannot be given with cisapride or astemazole.

serotonin selective reuptake inhibitors; sympathomimetic agents). The risk of hypertensive crisis and the hassle of restricting diet and medications have generally been the price that a patient has had to pay for the therapeutic benefits of the MAO inhibitors.

In the case of MAO B inhibitors, no significant amount of MAO A is inhibited, and there is very little risk of hypertension from dietary amines. Patients taking MAO B inhibitors to prevent progression of Parkinson's disease, for example, do not require any special diet. On the other hand, MAO B inhibitors are not effective antidepressants at doses that are selective for MAO B.

A newer class of MAO inhibitors, which has entered clinical practice for the treatment of depression, is known as reversible inhibitors of MAO A (RIMAs). This is a very welcome development in new drug therapeutics for depression, because it has the potential of making MAO A inhibition for the treatment of depression much safer. That is, the "suicide inhibitors" are associated with the dangerous hypertensive episodes mentioned above, which are caused when patients eat food rich in tyramine (such as cheese). This so-called cheese reaction occurs when the tyramine in the diet releases norepinephrine and other sympathomimetic amines (Fig. 1–23). When MAO is inhibited irreversibly, the levels of these amines rise to a dangerous level

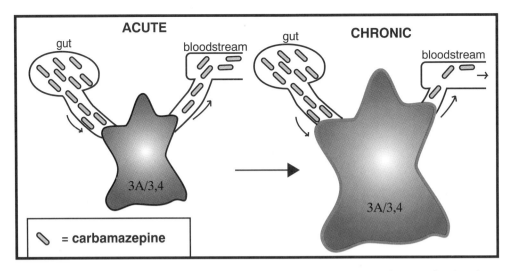

FIGURE 2–19. The anticonvulsant and mood stabilizer carbamazepine is a **substrate** for CYP450 **3A4**. It can also **induce** the metabolism of 3A4 by inducing more copies of the enzyme to be formed, thereby raising the enzyme activity of 3A4. Over time, therefore, carbamazepine doses may need to be increased to compensate for this increased metabolism.

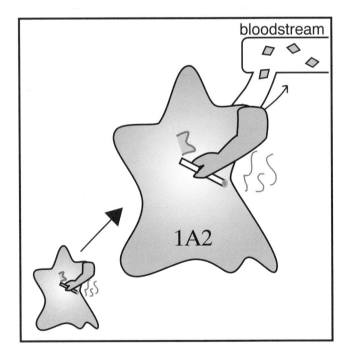

FIGURE 2–20. **Smoking** can **induce** the activity of CYP450 **1A2**. This might require that 1A2 substrates administered to a smoker be given in a higher dose. It may also require such 1A2 substrates to have their doses decreased if a smoker stops smoking.

Table 2–2. *Inhibition potential of antidepressants at CYP450 enzyme systems*

Relative rank	1A2	2C9/19	2D6	3A4
High	fluvoxamine	fluvoxamine fluoxetine	paroxetine fluoxetine	fluvoxamine nefazodone fluoxetine
Moderate to low	tertiary TCAs fluoxetine paroxetine	sertraline fluoxetine	secondary TCAs	sertraline TCAs paroxetine
Low to minimal	venlafaxine bupropion citalopram reboxetine mirtazapine sertraline nefazodone	venlafaxine bupropion citalopram reboxetine mirtazapine nefazodone paroxetine	venlafaxine bupropion citalopram reboxetine mirtazapine sertraline nefazodone fluvoxamine	venlafaxine bupropion citalopram reboxetine mirtazapine

Table 2–3. *Pharmacokinetics summary*

A few combinations must be avoided.
Several combinations require dosage adjustment of one of the drugs.
Many drug interactions are statistically significant but clinically insignificant.

Table 2–4. *Monoamine oxidase (MAO) inhibitors*

Classical MAO inhibitors—irreversible and nonselective
    phenelzine (Nardil)
    tranylcypromine (Parnate)
    isocarboxazid (Marplan)
Reversible inhibitors of MAO A (RIMAS)
    moclobemide (Aurorix)
Selective inhibitors of MAO B
    deprenyl (Selegiline; Eldepryl)

because they are not being destroyed by MAO. Blood pressure soars, even causing blood vessels to rupture in the brain.

Enter the reversible MAO inhibitors. If someone eats cheese, tyramine will still release sympathomimetic amines, but these amines will chase the reversible inhibitor off the MAO enzyme, allowing the dangerous amines to be destroyed (Fig. 2–24). This is sort of like having your cake—or cheese—and eating it, too. The reversible MAO inhibitors have the same therapeutic effects as the suicide inhibitors of MAO, but without the likelihood of a cheese reaction if a patient inadvertently takes in otherwise dangerous dietary tyramine.

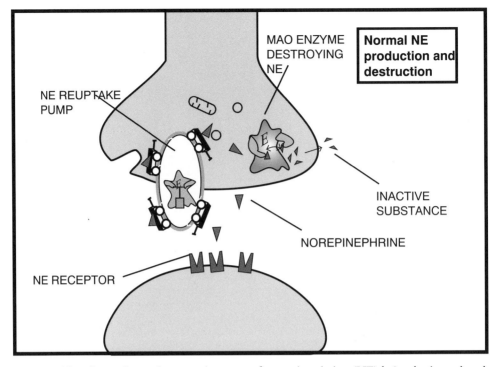

FIGURE 2–21. This figure shows the normal process of **norepinephrine (NE)** being both produced and **destroyed. Monoamine oxidase (MAO)** is the enzyme that normally acts to destroy NE to keep it in balance.

As MAO inhibitors have applications as second-line treatment for anxiety disorders, such as panic disorder and social phobia, in addition to depression, the RIMAs have the potential to make the treatment of these additional disorders by MAO A inhibition much safer as well.

In terms of the new MAO inhibitors that may become available in the future, it is possible that some new RIMAs may be approved as antidepressants. Moclobemide, available in many countries, is unlikely, for commercial reasons, to become available in the United States. Another promising RIMA, brofaramine, is also unlikely to be developed for any country. However, befloxatone is progressing in clinical trials, and other RIMAs are also potential drug development candidates, including RS-8359, cimoxatone, and toloxatone.

Tricyclic Antidepressants

The tricyclic antidepressants (Table 2–5) were so named because their organic chemical structure contains three rings (Fig. 2–25). The tricyclic antidepressants were synthesized about the same time as other three-ringed molecules that were shown to be effective tranquilizers for schizophrenia (i.e., the early antipsychotic neuroleptic drugs such as chlorpromazine) (Fig. 2–26). The tricyclic antidepressants were a disappointment when tested as antipsychotics. Even though they have a three-ringed structure, they were not effective in the treatment of schizophrenia and were almost

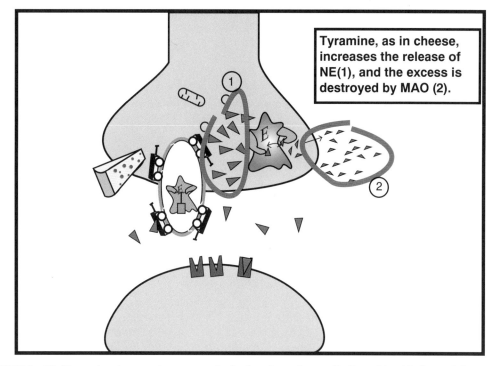

Tyramine, as in cheese, increases the release of NE(1), and the excess is destroyed by MAO (2).

FIGURE 2–22. **Tyramine** is an amine present in food such as **cheese**. Indicated in this figure is how tyramine (depicted as cheese) acts to **increase the release of norepinephrine (NE)** (red circle 1). However, in normal circumstances, the enzyme **monoamine oxidase (MAO) readily destroys the excess NE** released by tyramine, and no harm is done (see red circle 2).

discarded. However, during testing for schizophrenia, they were discovered to be antidepressants. That is, careful clinicians detected antidepressant properties, although not antipsychotic properties, in the schizophrenic patients. Thus, the antidepressant properties of the tricyclic antidepressants were serendipitously observed in the 1950s and 1960s, and eventually these compounds were marketed for the treatment of depression.

Long after their antidepressant properties were observed, the tricyclics were discovered to block the reuptake pumps for both serotonin and norepinephrine, and to a lesser extent, dopamine (Figs. 1–16, 2–5, and 2–6). Some tricyclics have more potency for inhibition of the serotonin reuptake pump (e.g., clomipramine); others are more selective for norepinephrine over serotonin (e.g., desipramine, maprotilene, nortriptyline, protriptyline). Most, however, block both serotonin and norepinephrine reuptake.

In addition, essentially all the tricyclic antidepressants have at least three other actions: blockade of muscarinic cholinergic receptors, blockade of H1 histamine receptors, and blockade of alpha 1 adrenergic receptors (Fig. 2–27). Whereas blockade of the serotonin and norepinephrine reuptake pumps is thought to account for the *therapeutic actions* of these drugs (Figs. 2–28 and 2–29), the other three pharmacologic properties are thought to account for their *side effects* (Figs. 2–30, 2–31, and

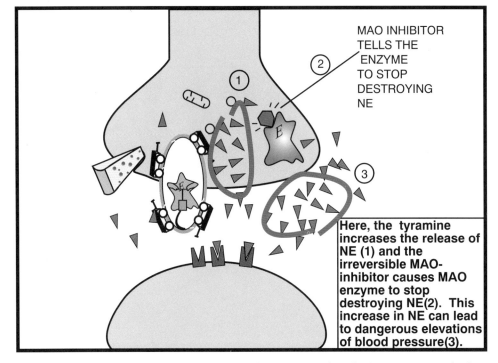

FIGURE 2–23. Here, tyramine is releasing norepinephrine (NE) (red circle 1) just as previously shown in Figure 2–9. However, this time **monoamine oxidase (MAO)** is also being **inhibited** by a typical, irreversible MAO inhibitor. This results in MAO **stopping its destruction of norepinephrine (NE)** (arrow 2). As already indicated in Figure 2–3, such MAO inhibition in itself causes **accumulation of NE**. However, when MAO inhibition is taking place in the presence of tyramine, the combination can lead to a very large accumulation of NE (red circle 3). Such a great NE accumulation can cause dangerous elevations of blood pressure.

2–32). Some of the tricyclic antidepressants also have the ability to block serotonin 2A receptors, which may contribute to the therapeutic actions of those agents with this property. Blockade of serotonin 2A receptors is discussed in Chapter 3. Tricyclic antidepressants also block sodium channels in the heart and brain, which can cause cardiac arrhythmias and cardiac arrest in overdose, as well as seizures.

In terms of the *therapeutic actions* of tricyclic antidepressants, they essentially work as allosteric modulators of the neurotransmitter reuptake process. Specifically, they are negative allosteric modulators. After the neurotransmitter norepinephrine or serotonin binds to its own selective receptor site, it is normally transported back into the presynaptic neuron as discussed in Chapter 1 (Fig. 1–16). However, when certain antidepressants bind to an allosteric site close to the neurotransmitter transporter, this causes the neurotransmitter to no longer be able to bind there, thus blocking synaptic reuptake of the neurotransmitter (Figs. 2–28 and 2–29). Therefore, norepinephrine and serotonin cannot be shuttled back into the presynaptic neuron.

In terms of side effects of the tricyclic antidepressants (Table 2–5), blockade of alpha 1 adrenergic receptors causes orthostatic hypotension and dizziness (Fig. 2–30). Anticholinergic actions at muscarinic cholinergic receptors cause dry mouth, blurred vision, urinary retention, and constipation and memory disturbances (Fig.

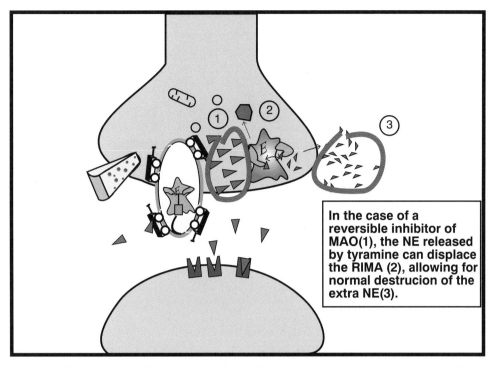

In the case of a reversible inhibitor of MAO(1), the NE released by tyramine can displace the RIMA (2), allowing for normal destrucion of the extra NE(3).

FIGURE 2–24. Shown in this figure also is the **combination of a monoamine oxidase (MAO) inhibitor and tyramine**. However, in this case the MAO inhibitor is of the **reversible** type (reversible inhibitor of MAO A, or **RIMA**). In contrast to the situation shown in the previous figure (Fig. 2–23), the accumulation of norepinephrine (NE) caused by tyramine (indicated in red circle 1) can actually strip the RIMA off MAO (arrow 2). MAO, now devoid of its inhibitor, can merrily do its job, which is to destroy the NE (red circle 3) and thus prevent the dangerous accumulation of NE. Such a reversal of MAO by NE is only possible with a RIMA and not with the classical MAO inhibitors, which are completely irreversible.

Table 2–5. *Tricyclic antidepressants*

clomipramine (Anafranil)
imipramine (Tofranil)
amitriptyline (Elavil; Endep; Tryptizol; Loroxyl)
nortriptyline (Pamelor; Noratren)
protriptyline (Vivactil)
maprotiline (Ludiomil)
amoxapine (Asendin)
doxepin (Sinequan; Adapin)
desipramine (Norpramin; Pertofran)
trimipramine (Surmontil)

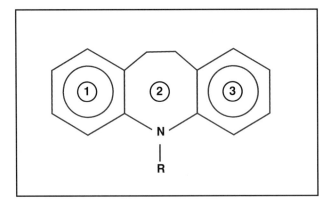

FIGURE 2–25. This is the **chemical structure of a tricyclic antidepressant (TCA)**. The three rings show how this group of drugs got its name.

2–31). Blockade of H1 histamine receptors causes sedation and weight gain (Fig. 2–32).

The term *tricyclic antidepressant* is archaic by today's pharmacology. First, the antidepressants that block biogenic amine reuptake are no longer all tricyclic; the new agents can have one, two, three, or four rings in their structures. Second, the tricyclic antidepressants are not merely antidepressant since some of them have anti-obsessive compulsive disorder effects and others have antipanic effects.

Like the MAO inhibitors, tricyclic antidepressants have fallen into second-line use for depression in North America and much of Europe. However, there still remains considerable use of these agents, and they are even among the most frequently prescribed antidepressants in certain countries, including Germany and countries in Latin America, as well as in the Third World, where generic pricing makes these agents less expensive than the newer antidepressants that are still under patent protection.

Selective Serotonin Reuptake Inhibitors

What Five Drugs Share in Common

The SSRIs comprise a class of drugs with five prominent members, which together account for the majority of prescriptions for antidepressants in the United States and several other countries. These are fluoxetine, sertraline, paroxetine, fluvoxamine, and citalopram (Table 2–6). Although each of these five SSRIs belongs to a chemically distinct family, all have a single major pharmacologic feature in common, namely, selective and potent inhibition of serotonin reuptake, which is more powerful than their actions on norepinephrine reuptake or on alpha 1, histamine 1, or muscarinic cholinergic receptors, and with virtually no ability to block sodium channels, even in overdose. This simple concept is shown in Figs. 2–33 and 2–34.

Thus, the SSRIs all share important differentiating features from the tricyclic antidepressants, which they have largely replaced in clinical practice. That is, SSRIs have more powerful and selective serotonin reuptake inhibiting properties than the tricyclic antidepressants. By removing undesirable pharmacologic properties of the

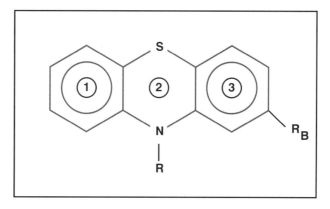

FIGURE 2–26. This is a general **chemical formula for the phenothiazine type of antipsychotic drugs**. These drugs also have three rings, and the first antidepressants were modeled after such drugs.

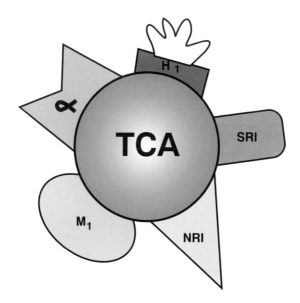

The **Tricyclic Antidepressant** has five actions:
blocking the reuptake of serotonin, blocking the reuptake
of norepinephrine, blockade of alpha 1 adrenergic
receptors, blockade of H1 histamine receptors,
and blockade of muscarinic cholinergic receptors.

FIGURE 2–27. Shown here is an icon of a **tricyclic antidepressant (TCA)**. These drugs are actually **five drugs in one:** (1) a serotonin reuptake inhibitor (SRI); (2) a norepinephrine reuptake inhibitor (NRI); (3) an anticholinergic/antimuscarinic drug (M1); (4) an alpha adrenergic antagonist (alpha); and (5) an antihistamine (H1).

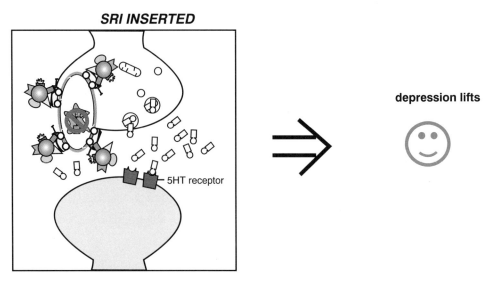

FIGURE 2–28. **Therapeutic actions of the tricyclic antidepressants—part 1.** In this diagram, the icon of the **TCA** is shown with its serotonin reuptake inhibitor (**SRI**) portion inserted into the serotonin reuptake pump, blocking it and causing an **antidepressant effect**.

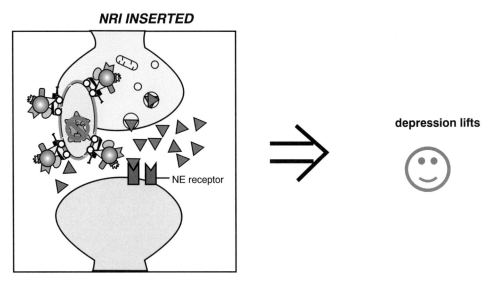

FIGURE 2–29. **Therapeutic actions of the tricyclic antidepressants—part 2.** In this diagram, the icon of the **TCA** is shown with its norepinephrine reuptake inhibitor (**NRI**) portion inserted into the norepinephrine reuptake pump, blocking it and causing an **antidepressant effect**. Thus, both the serotonin reuptake portion (see Fig. 2–28) and the NRI portion of the TCA act pharmacologically to cause an antidepressant effect.

90

H1 INSERTED

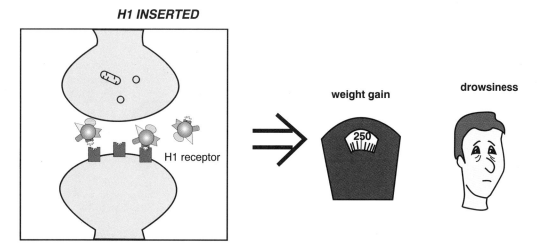

FIGURE 2–30. *Side effects of the tricyclic antidepressants*—part 1. In this diagram, the icon of the **TCA** is shown with its antihistamine (**H1**) portion inserted into histamine receptors, causing the side effects of **weight gain and drowsiness**.

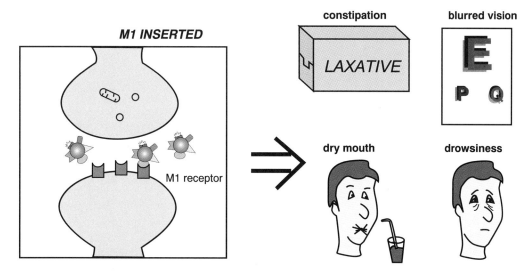

FIGURE 2–31. *Side effects of the tricyclic antidepressants*—part 2. In this diagram, the icon of the **TCA** is shown with its anticholinergic/antimuscarinic (M1) portion inserted into acetylcholine receptors, causing the side effects of **constipation, blurred vision, dry mouth, and drowsiness**.

tricyclics, the SSRIs also eliminated the undesirable side effects associated with them (Figs. 2–30 to 2–32). In particular, SSRIs lack the danger in overdose that the tricyclics all share. Whereas a 15-day supply of a tricyclic antidepressant can be a lethal dose, SSRIs, by contrast, rarely if ever cause death in overdose by themselves.

Pharmacologic and Molecular Mechanism of Action of the SSRIs

Although the action of SSRIs at the *presynaptic axon terminal* has classically been emphasized (Figs. 2–1 through 2–6), research has more recently determined that

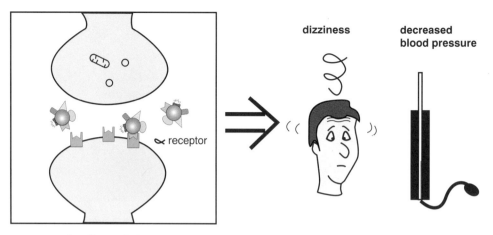

dizziness

decreased blood pressure

α receptor

FIGURE 2–32. *Side effects of the tricyclic antidepressants*—part 3. In this diagram, the icon of the **TCA** is shown with its alpha adrenergic antagonist (alpha) portion inserted into alpha adrenergic receptors, causing the side effects of **dizziness, decreased blood pressure, and drowsiness.**

Table 2–6. *Serotonin selective reuptake inhibitors (SSRIs)*

fluoxetine (Prozac)
sertraline (Zoloft)
paroxetine (Paxil)
fluvoxamine (Luvox, Feverin, Dumirox, Floxyfral)
citalopram (Celexa, Cipramil, Serostat, Cipram)

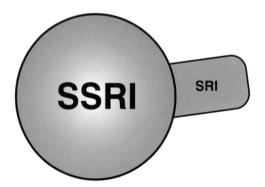

FIGURE 2–33. Shown here is the icon of a selective **serotonin** reuptake inhibitor (**SSRI**). In this case, four of the five pharmacological properties of the tricyclic antidepressants (TCAs) (Fig. 2–27) were removed. Only the serotonin reuptake inhibitor (**SRI**) portion remains; thus the SRI action is selective, which is why these agents are called **selective SRIs.**

SSRI ACTION

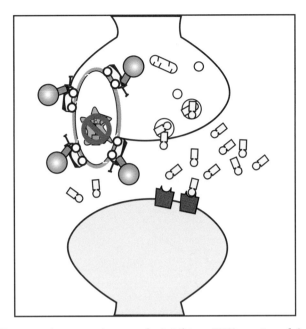

FIGURE 2–34. In this diagram, the serotonin reuptake inhibitor (**SRI**) portion of the **SSRI** molecule is shown inserted into the serotonin reuptake pump, blocking it and causing an **antidepressant effect**. This is analogous to one of the dimensions of the tricyclic antidepressants (TCAs), already shown in Figure 2–28.

events occurring at the *somatodendritic* end of the serotonin neuron (near the cell body) may be more important in explaining their therapeutic actions (Figs. 2–35 through 2–38). It may be that the events occurring at postsynaptic serotonin neurons mediate the acute side effects and the development of tolerance to these side effects over time (Fig. 2–39).

The monoamine hypothesis of depression states that in the depressed state (Fig. 2–35), serotonin may be deficient, both at presynaptic somatodendritic areas near the cell body and in the synapse itself near the axon terminal. Neuronal firing rates may be diminished. Also, the neurotransmitter receptor hypothesis states that pre- and postsynaptic receptors may be up-regulated. The monoamine hypothesis of delayed gene action suggests that these receptors may not be able to transduce receptor occupancy by serotonin into the necessary regulation of postsynaptic genes, such as those for the neurotrophic factor BDNF (see Figs. 1–63 and 2–7). These ideas are shown in Figure 2–35 and may be the starting point for the serotonin neuron and its targets when SSRIs are first administered to a depressed patient. On the other hand, it is also possible that the serotonin neuron is actually normal but that the events triggered by SSRIs compensate for neurochemical deficiencies elsewhere in the brain.

When an SSRI is given acutely, serotonin rises owing to blockade of its transport pump. What was surprising to discover, however, is that blocking the presynaptic reuptake pump does *not* immediately lead to a great deal of serotonin in the synapse.

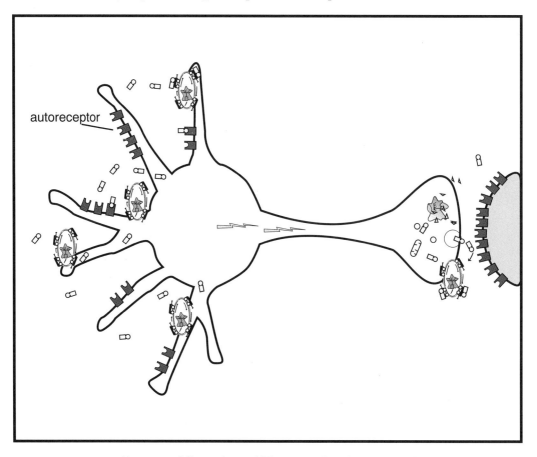

Depressed State: Low 5HT, up-regulated receptors, low amount of signals in the neuron to release more 5HT

FIGURE 2–35. *Mechanism of action of serotonin selective reuptake inhibitors (SSRIs)*—part 1. Depicted here is a **serotonin neuron in a depressed patient**. In depression, the serotonin neuron is conceptualized as having a relative **deficiency of the neurotransmitter serotonin**. Also, the number of **serotonin receptors** is **up-regulated**, or increased, including presynaptic **autoreceptors** as well as **postsynaptic receptors**.

In fact, when SSRI treatment is initiated, 5HT rises to a much higher level at the cell body area in the midbrain raphe than in the areas of the brain where the axons terminate (Fig. 2–36). The somatodendritic area of the serotonin neuron is where the serotonin (5HT) first increases, and the serotonin receptors there have 5HT1A pharmacology. Such immediate pharmacologic actions obviously cannot explain the delayed therapeutic actions of the SSRIs. However, these immediate actions may explain the side effects that are caused by the SSRIs when treatment is initiated.

Over time, the increased 5HT at the somatodendritic 5HT1A autoreceptors causes them to down-regulate and become desensitized (Fig. 2–37). When the increase in serotonin is recognized by these presynaptic 5HT1A receptors, this information is sent to the cell nucleus of the serotonin neuron. The genome's reaction to this information is to issue instructions that cause these same receptors to become de-

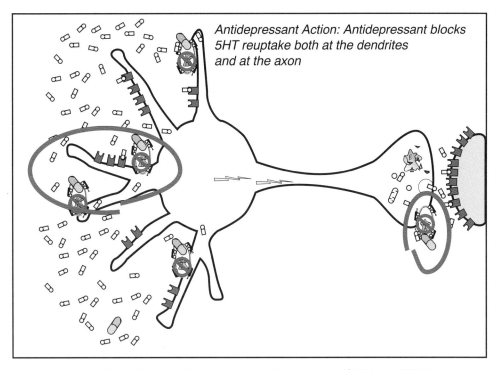

FIGURE 2–36. *Mechanism of action of serotonin selective reuptake inhibitors (SSRIs)*—part 2. When an SSRI is administered, it immediately blocks the serotonin reuptake pump (see icon of an SSRI drug capsule blocking the reuptake pump). However, this causes **serotonin to increase initially only in the somatodendritic area** of the serotonin neuron (left) and not in the axon terminals (right).

sensitized over time. The time course of this desensitization correlates with the onset of the therapeutic actions of the SSRIs.

Once the 5HT1A somatodendritic autoreceptors are desensitized, 5HT can no longer effectively inhibit its own release, and the serotonin neuron is therefore disinhibited. This results in a flurry of 5HT release from axons due to an increase in neuronal impulse flow (Fig. 2–38). This is just another way of saying that the serotonin release is "turned on" at the axon terminals. The serotonin that now pours out of the various projections of serotonin pathways in the brain theoretically mediates the various therapeutic actions of the SSRIs.

While the presynaptic somatodendritic 5HT1A autoreceptors are desensitizing, serotonin is building up in synapses, causing the postsynaptic serotonin receptors to desensitize as well. This happens because the increase in synaptic serotonin is recognized by postsynaptic serotonin 2A, 2C, 3, and other receptors. These receptors in turn send this information to the cell nucleus of the *postsynaptic* neuron that serotonin is targeting. The reaction of the genome in the postsynaptic neuron is also to issue instructions to down-regulate or desensitize these receptors. The time course of this desensitization correlates with the onset of tolerance to the side effects of the SSRIs (Fig. 2–39).

This theory thus suggests a pharmacological cascading mechanism, whereby the SSRIs exert their therapeutic actions, namely, powerful disinhibition of serotonin

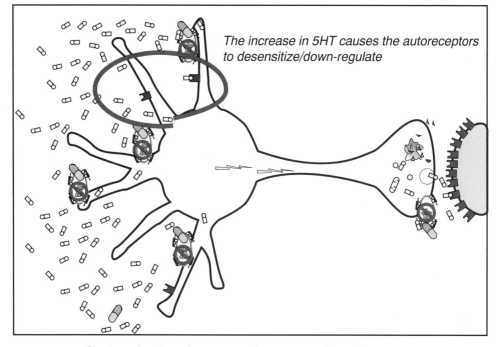

The increase in 5HT causes the autoreceptors to desensitize/down-regulate

FIGURE 2–37. *Mechanism of action of serotonin selective reuptake inhibitors (SSRIs)*—part 3. The consequence of serotonin increasing in the somatodentritic area of the serotonin neuron, as depicted in the Figure 2–36, is to cause the **somatodendritic serotonin 1A autoreceptors to desensitize or down-regulate** (red circle).

release in key pathways throughout the brain. Furthermore, side effects are hypothetically caused by the acute actions of serotonin at undesirable receptors in undesirable pathways. Finally, side effects may attenuate over time by desensitization of the very receptors that mediate them.

There are potentially exciting corollaries to this hypothesis. First, if the ultimate increase in serotonin at critical synapses is required for therapeutic actions, then its failure to occur may explain why some patients respond to an SSRI and others do not. Also, if new drugs could be designed to increase serotonin at the right places at a faster rate, it could result in a much needed rapid-acting antidepressant. Such ideas are mere research hypotheses at this time but could lead to additional studies clarifying the molecular events that are key mediators of depressive illness as well as of antidepressant treatment responses.

Serotonin Pathways and Receptors That Mediate Therapeutic Actions and Side Effects of SSRIs

As mentioned above, the SSRIs cause both their therapeutic actions and their side effects by increasing serotonin at synapses, where reuptake is blocked and serotonin release is disinhibited. In general, increasing serotonin in desirable pathways and at targeted receptor subtypes leads to the well-known therapeutic actions of these drugs. However, since SSRIs increase serotonin in virtually every serotonin pathway

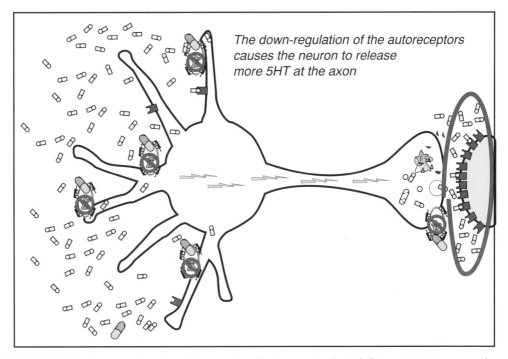

The down-regulation of the autoreceptors causes the neuron to release more 5HT at the axon

FIGURE 2–38. *Mechanism of action of serotonin selective reuptake inhibitors (SSRIs)*—part 4. Once the somatodendritic autoreceptors down-regulate as depicted in Figure 2–37, there is no longer inhibition of impulse flow in the serotonin neuron. Thus, **neuronal impulse flow is turned on**. The consequence of this is **release of serotonin in the axon terminal** (red circle). However, **this increase is delayed** as compared with the increase of serotonin in the somatodendritic areas of the serotonin neuron, depicted in Figure 2–36. This delay is the result of the time it takes for somatodendritic serotonin to down-regulate the serotonin 1A autoreceptors and turn on neuronal impulse flow in the serotonin neuron. This delay may explain why antidepressants do not relieve depression immediately. It is also the reason why the mechanism of action of antidepressants may be linked to increasing neuronal impulse flow in serotonin neurons, with serotonin levels increasing at axon terminals before an SSRI can exert its antidepressant effects.

and at virtually every serotonin receptor, some of these serotonin actions are undesirable and therefore account for side effects. By understanding the functions of the various serotonin pathways and the distribution of the various serotonin receptor subtypes, it is possible to gain insight into both the therapeutic actions and the side effects that the SSRIs share as a class.

In terms of antidepressant actions, evidence points to the projection of serotonin neurons from the midbrain raphe to frontal cortex as the substrate of this therapeutic action (Fig. 1–51). Therapeutic actions in bulimia, binge eating, and various other eating disorders may be mediated by serotonin's pathway from raphe to hypothalamic feeding and appetite centers (Fig. 1–55).

Because different pathways seem to mediate the different therapeutic actions of SSRIs, it would not be surprising if serotonin's therapeutic roles differed from one therapeutic indication to another. This, indeed, seems to be the case and may be the basis for the different therapeutic profiles of SSRIs from one therapeutic indication to another. Contrasting antidepressant and antibulimic actions, for example, are in-

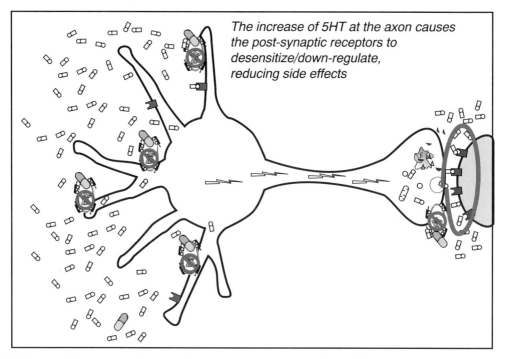

The increase of 5HT at the axon causes the post-synaptic receptors to desensitize/down-regulate, reducing side effects

FIGURE 2–39. *Mechanism of action of serotonin selective reuptake inhibitors (SSRIs)*—part 5. Finally, once the SSRIs have blocked the reuptake pump (Fig. 2–36), increased somatodendritic serotonin (Fig. 2–36), desensitized somatodendritic serotonin 1A autoreceptors (Fig. 2–37), turned on neuronal impulse flow (Fig. 2–38), and increased release of serotonin from axon terminals (Fig. 2–38), the final step shown here may be the desensitization of postsynaptic serotonin receptors. This has also been shown in previous figures demonstrating the actions of monoamine oxidase (MAO) inhibitors (Fig. 2–4) and the actions of tricyclic antidepressants (Fig. 2–6). This desensitization may mediate the reduction of side effects of SSRIs as tolerance develops.

Table 2–7. *Antidepressant profile of SSRIs*

Starting dose usually the same as the maintenance dose
Onset of response usually 3 to 8 weeks
Response is frequently complete remission of symptoms
Target symptoms do not worsen when treatment initiated

dicated by differing doses, onsets of action, and documentation of long-term actions, as summarized in Tables 2–7 and 2–8.

In terms of side effects of SSRIs, acute stimulation of at least four serotonin receptor subtypes may be responsible for mediating these undesirable actions. These include the 5HT2A, 5HT2C, 5HT3, and 5HT4 receptors. Since SSRI side effects are generally acute, starting from the first dose and if anything attenuate over time, it may be that the acute increase in synaptic serotonin is sufficient to mediate side effects but insufficient to mediate therapeutic effects until the much more robust disinhibition of the neuron "kicks in" once autoreceptors are down regulated. If the

Table 2-8. *Antibulimic profile of SSRIs*

Usual starting dose is higher than for other indications
Onset of response may be faster than for other indications
May not be as effective as for other indications in maintaining acute effects chronically
Fluoxetine has best efficacy data to date and also serotonin 2C properties
Target symptoms do not worsen on initiation of treatment

postsynaptic receptors that theoretically mediate side effects down regulate or desensitize, the side effects attenuate or go away. Presumably, the signal of receptor occupancy of serotonin to the postsynaptic receptor is detected by the genome of the target neuron, and decreasing the genetic expression of these receptors that mediate the side effects causes the side effects to go away.

The undesirable side effects of SSRIs seem to involve not only specific serotonin receptor subtypes but also the action of serotonin at the receptors in specific areas of the body, including brain, spinal cord, and gut. The topography of serotonin receptor subtypes in different serotonin pathways may thus help to explain how side effects are mediated. Thus, acute stimulation of serotonin 2A and 2C receptors in the projection from raphe to limbic cortex may cause the acute mental agitation, anxiety, or induction of panic attacks that can be observed with early dosing of an SSRI (Fig. 1–54). Acute stimulation of the 2A receptors in the basal ganglia may lead to changes in motor movements due to serotonin's inhibition of dopamine neurotransmission there (Fig. 1–53). Thus, akathisia (restlessness), psychomotor retardation, or even mild parkinsonism and dystonic movements can result. Stimulation of serotonin 2A receptors in the brainstem sleep centers may cause rapid muscle movements called *myoclonus* during the night; it may also disrupt slow-wave sleep and cause nocturnal awakenings (Fig. 1–56). Stimulation of serotonin 2A receptors in the spinal cord may inhibit the spinal reflexes of orgasm and ejaculation and cause sexual dysfunction (Fig. 1–57). Stimulation of serotonin 2A receptors in mesocortical pleasure centers may reduce dopamine activity there and cause apathy (e.g., apathetic recoveries discussed in Chapter 1; see Table 1–18) or decreased libido.

Stimulation of serotonin 3 receptors in the hypothalamus or brainstem may cause nausea or vomiting, respectively (Fig. 1–58). Stimulation of serotonin 3 and 4 receptors in the gastrointestinal tract may cause increased bowel motility, gastrointestinal cramps and diarrhea (Fig. 1–59).

Thus, virtually all side effects of the SSRIs can be understood as undesirable actions of serotonin in undesirable pathways at undesirable receptor subtypes. This appears to be the "cost of doing business," as it is not possible for a systemically administered SSRI to act only at the desirable receptors in the desirable places; it must act everywhere it is distributed, which means all over the brain and all over the body. Fortunately, SSRI side effects are more of a nuisance than a danger, and they generally attenuate over time, although they can cause an important subset of patients to discontinue an SSRI prematurely.

Although several SSRIs other than the five listed in Table 2–6 have been synthesized, with the exception of the active enantiomers of currently marketed SSRIs such as fluoxetine and citalopram, it is unlikely any new SSRI will be developed as an antidepressant, as many other novel mechanisms are now available for clinical testing. Extended-release formulations of currently marketed SSRIs such as paroxetine and fluvoxamine may also become available. One novel and distinct mechanism related to the SSRIs is exemplified by tianeptine. This agent is in clinical testing and available in France as a counterintuitive serotonin reuptake *enhancer*. Whether this will develop into a well-documented antidepressant worldwide is still unknown.

Not-So-Selective Serotonin Reuptake Inhibitors: Five Unique Drugs or One Class with Five Members?

Although the SSRIs clearly share the same mechanism of action, therapeutic profiles, and overall side effect profiles, individual patients often react very differently to one SSRI versus another. This is not generally observed in large clinical trials, where group differences between two SSRIs either in efficacy or in side effects are very difficult to document. Rather, such differences are seen by prescribers treating patients one at a time, with some patients experiencing a therapeutic response to one SSRI and not another and other patients tolerating one SSRI but not another.

Although there is no generally accepted explanation that accounts for these commonly observed clinical phenomena, it makes sense to consider the pharmacologic characteristics of the five SSRIs that differ one from another as candidates for explaining the broad range of individual patient reactions to different SSRIs. Now that the SSRIs have been in widespread clinical use for over a decade, pharmacologists have discovered that these five drugs have actions at receptors other than the serotonin transporter and at various enzymes that may be important to their overall actions, both therapeutically and in terms of tolerability.

The reality is that one or another of the SSRIs has pharmacologic actions within one or two orders of magnitude of their potencies for serotonin reuptake inhibition at a wide variety of receptors and enzymes. Furthermore, no two SSRIs have identical secondary pharmacological characteristics. These actions can include norepinephrine reuptake blockade, dopamine reuptake blockade, serotonin 2C agonist actions, muscarinic cholinergic antagonist actions, interaction with the sigma receptor, inhibition of the enzyme nitric oxide synthetase, and inhibition of the cytochrome P450 enzymes 1A2, 2D6, and 3A4 (Fig. 2–40). Whether these secondary binding profiles can account for the differences in efficacy and tolerability in individual patients remains to be proved. However, it does lead to provocative hypothesis generation and gives a rational basis for physicians not to be denied access to one or another of the SSRIs by payors claiming "they are all the same."

The candidate secondary pharmacologic mechanisms for each of the five SSRIs are shown in Figures 2–41 to 2–45. These may lead to variations from one drug to another that could prove potentially more advantageous or less advantageous for different patient profiles. However, these are hypotheses that as yet are unconfirmed. Nevertheless, there are real differences among the five SSRIs for many individual patients, and sometimes only an empirical trial of different SSRIs will lead to the best match of a drug to an individual patient.

Selective Noradrenergic Reuptake Inhibitors

Although some tricyclic antidepressants (e.g., desipramine, maprotilene) block norepinephrine reuptake more potently than serotonin reuptake, even these tricyclics

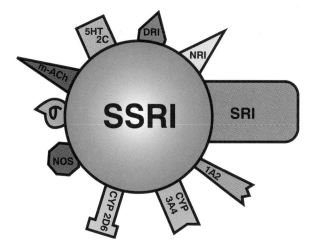

FIGURE 2–40. Icon of various **secondary pharmacologic properties** that may be associated with one or more of the five different **SSRIs**. This includes not only serotonin reuptake inhibition (SRI), but also lesser degrees of actions at other neurotransmitter receptors and enzymes, including norepinephrine reuptake inhibition (NRI), dopamine reuptake inhibition (DRI), serotonin 2C agonist actions (5HT2C), muscarinic/cholinergic antagonist actions (m-ACH), sigma actions (sigma), and inhibition of nitric oxide synthetase (NOS), CYP450 2D6, 3A4, or 1A2.

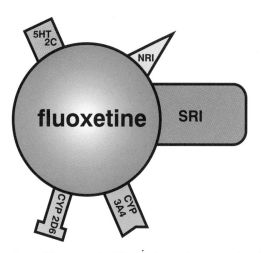

FIGURE 2–41. Icon of **fluoxetine** with serotonin 2C agonist action, norepinephrine reuptake inhibition (NRI), and 2D6 and 3A4 inhibition, in addition to serotonin reuptake inhibition (SRI).

are not really selective, since they still block alpha 1, histamine 1, and muscarinic cholinergic receptors, as do all tricyclics. The first truly selective noradrenergic reuptake inhibitor (NRI) is reboxetine, which lacks these undesirable binding properties (Figs. 2–46 and 2–47).

Thus, reboxetine is the logical pharmacological complement to the SSRIs—since it provides selective *noradrenergic* reuptake inhibition greater than serotonin reuptake inhibition but without the undesirable binding properties of the tricyclic antidepressants. The discovery of reboxetine has given rise to the questions: What is the

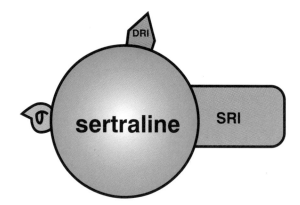

FIGURE 2–42. Icon of **sertraline** with dopamine reuptake inhibition (DRI) and sigma actions, in addition to serotonin reuptake inhibition (SRI).

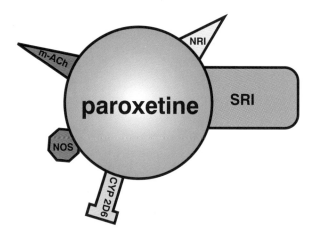

FIGURE 2–43. Icon of **paroxetine** with muscarinic/cholinergic antagonist actions (mACH), norepinephrine reuptake inhibition (NRI), and serotonin 2D6 and 3A4 inhibition, in addition to serotonin reuptake inhibition (SRI).

clinical difference between increasing noradrenergic neurotransmission and increasing serotonergic neurotransmission? Since norepinephrine and serotonin are intimately interrelated, does it make any difference which reuptake pump is inhibited?

Although norepinephrine and serotonin have overlapping functions in the regulation of mood, the hypothetical noradrenaline deficiency syndrome is not identical to the hypothetical serotonin deficiency syndrome (Tables 1–21 and 1–23). Furthermore, not all patients with depression respond to an SSRI nor do all respond to a selective NRI, although more may respond to agents or combinations of agents that block both serotonin and norepinephrine reuptake. Moreover, many patients who respond to serotonin reuptake blockers do not remit completely and seem to have improved mood but an enduring noradrenergic deficiency syndrome, which is sometimes called an apathetic response to the SSRI (e.g., Table 1–18).

Although it is not yet possible to determine who will respond to a serotonergic agent and who to a noradrenergic agent prior to empirical treatment, there is the

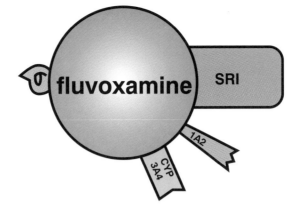

FIGURE 2–44. Icon of **fluvoxamine** with sigma actions and serotonin 1A2 and 3A4 inhibition, in addition to serotonin reuptake inhibition (SRI).

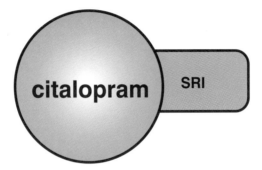

FIGURE 2–45. Icon of **citalopram**, relatively selective for serotonin reuptake inhibition (SRI).

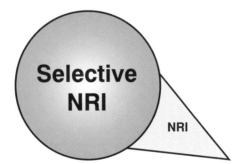

FIGURE 2–46. Icon of a **selective norepinephrine reuptake inhibitor** (NRI).

notion that those with the serotonin deficiency syndrome (i.e., depression associated with anxiety, panic, phobias, posttraumatic stress disorder, obsessions, compulsions, or eating disorders) might be more responsive to serotonergic antidepressants. This is supported by the fact that serotonergic antidepressants are efficacious not only in depression but also in obsessive-compulsive disorder, eating disorders, panic, social phobia, and even posttraumatic stress disorder, whereas noradrenergic antidepressants

Selective NRI ACTION

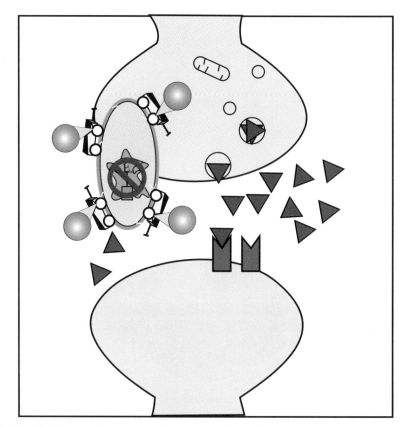

FIGURE 2–47. In this diagram, the norepinephrine reuptake inhibitor (**NRI**) portion of the selective NRI molecule is shown inserted in the norepinephrine reuptake pump, blocking it and causing an **antidepressant effect**.

are not well documented to improve generalized anxiety, panic, phobias, obsessive-compulsive disorder, or eating disorders.

On the other hand, patients with the noradrenergic deficiency syndrome (i.e., those whose depression is associated with fatigue, apathy, and notable cognitive disturbances, particularly impaired concentration, problems with sustaining and focusing attention, slowness in information processing, and deficiencies in working memory) may theoretically be more responsive to noradrenergic agents. Since the selective noradrenergic reuptake inhibitors have only recently become available, this theory is based on animal research. Confirmation of the usefulness of this approach in clinical practice awaits the results of ongoing research. Nevertheless, just as the SSRIs, first introduced for the treatment of depression, expanded their therapeutic uses to a host of anxiety disorders and other applications, so will the selective NRIs undoubtedly expand their therapeutic uses beyond the treatment of depression. For example, other theoretical considerations from preclinical work suggest that norad-

Table 2–9. *Potential therapeutic profile of reboxetine*

Depression
Fatigue
Apathy
Psychomotor retardation
Attention deficit and impaired concentration
Disorders (not limited to depression) characterized by cognitive slowing, especially
    deficiencies in working memory and in the speed of information processing

renergic enhancement should improve overall social functioning and work capacity by targeting psychomotor retardation, fatique, and apathy (Table 2–9). Noradrenergic enhancement might even boost cognitive functioning in disorders other than depression that are characterized by deficits in attention and memory, such as Alzheimer's disease, attention deficit disorder, and the cognitive disturbances associated with schizophrenia (Table 2–9).

Early indications from the use of reboxetine show that its efficacy is at least comparable to that of the tricyclic antidepressants and the SSRIs. In addition, reboxetine may specifically enhance social functioning, perhaps by converting apathetic responders into full remitters. Furthermore, reboxetine may be useful for severe depression, for depression unresponsive to other antidepressants, and as an adjunct to serotonergic antidepressants when dual neurotransmitter mechanisms are necessary to treat the most difficult cases.

Several specific noradrenergic pathways and receptors mediate both the therapeutic actions and the side effects of selective noradrenergic reuptake inhibitors (NRIs). As discussed above for the SSRIs, an analogous set of actions by norepinephrine in various noradrenergic pathways and at various noradrenergic receptors throughout the brain and the body may explain both the therapeutic actions and the side effects of the selective NRIs. That is, increasing norepinephrine at desirable synapses and at desirable noradrenergic receptors would lead to the therapeutic properties of the selective NRIs. Side effects would be due to increasing norepinephrine at undesirable places at the "cost of doing business," since selective NRIs increase norepinephrine in virtually every noradrenergic pathway and at virtually every noradrenergic receptor. By understanding the functions of the various norepinephrine pathways and the distribution of the various noradrenergic receptor subtypes, it is possible to gain insight into both the therapeutic actions and the side effects of the selective NRIs, such as reboxetine (Fig. 1–23).

In terms of antidepressant actions, evidence points to the projection of noradrenergic neurons from the locus coeruleus to the frontal cortex as the substrate of this therapeutic action (Fig. 1–24). The noradrenergic receptor subtype that may mediate norepinephrine's antidepressant actions there is the beta 1 postsynaptic receptor. Therapeutic actions in cognition are not yet established but could theoretically be mediated by norepinephrine's pathway from the locus coeruleus to other areas of the frontal cortex (Fig. 1–25). Postsynaptic receptors thought to mediate cognitive actions of norepinephrine in animal models are especially the alpha 2 noradrenergic receptor subtype. Therapeutic actions in improving apathy, fatigue, and psychomotor retardation could theoretically be mediated by the noradrenergic pathway from the locus coeruleus to the limbic cortex (Fig. 1–26).

Experience with the SSRIs predicts that as therapeutic actions of selective NRIs expand beyond antidepressant actions, the doses of drug, onsets of action, degrees of efficacy, and tolerability profiles may differ from one therapeutic use to another (Table 2–7 and 2–8).

In terms of side effects of the selective NRIs, acute stimulation of at least four clinically important noradrenergic receptor subtypes in various parts of the brain and body may be responsible for mediating these undesirable actions. This includes alpha 1 postsynaptic receptors, alpha 2 presynaptic receptors, alpha 2 postsynaptic receptors, and beta 1 postsynaptic noradrenergic receptors. As with the SSRIs, the side effects of selective NRIs are generally acute, starting from the first dose and if anything, attenuate over time. If the receptors that mediate side effects down regulate or desensitize, the side effects attenuate or go away.

Side effects of selective NRIs seem to involve not only specific noradrenergic receptor subtypes but also the action of norepinephrine at its receptors in specific areas of the body, including brain, spinal cord, heart, gastrointestinal tract, and urinary bladder. The topography of noradrenergic receptor subtypes in different nor-epinephrine pathways may thus help to explain how such side effects are mediated (Fig. 1–23). Thus, acute stimulation of beta 1 receptors in the cerebellum or pe-ripheral sympathetic nervous system may cause motor activation or tremor (Fig. 1–27). Acute stimulation of noradrenergic receptors in the limbic system may cause agitation (Fig. 1–26). Acute stimulation of noradrenergic receptors in the brainstem cardiovascular centers and descending into the spinal cord may alter blood pressure (Fig. 1–28).

Stimulation of beta 1 noradrenergic receptors in the heart may cause changes in heart rate (Fig. 1–29). Stimulation of noradrenergic receptors in the sympathetic nervous system may also cause a net reduction of parasympathetic cholinergic tone, since these systems often have reciprocal roles in peripheral organs and tissues. Thus, increased norepinephrine may produce symptoms reminiscent of anticholinergic side effects. This is not due to direct blockade of muscarinic cholinergic receptors but to indirect reduction of net parasympathetic tone resulting from increased sympathetic tone. Thus, a "pseudo-anticholinergic" syndrome of dry mouth, constipation, and urinary retention (Fig. 1–30) may be caused by selective NRIs, even though they have no direct actions on cholinergic receptors. Usually, however, the indirect re-duction of cholinergic tone yields milder and shorter lasting symptoms than does direct blockade of muscarinic cholinergic receptors.

Thus, virtually all side effects of the selective NRIs can be understood as unde-sirable actions of norepinephrine in undesirable pathways at undesirable receptor subtypes. Just as for the SSRIs, this occurs because it is not possible for a systemically administered drug to act only at the desirable receptors in the desirable places; it must act everywhere it is distributed, which means all over the brain and all over the body. Fortunately, selective NRI side effects are more of a nuisance than a danger, and they generally attenuate over time, although they can cause an important subset of patients to discontinue treatment.

In addition to reboxetine, which is currently marketed, other selective NRIs are in clinical testing at present for depression or attention deficit disorder. These include

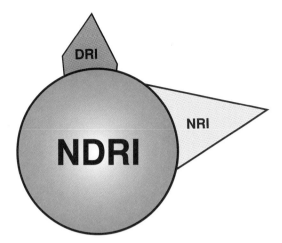

FIGURE 2–48. Shown here is the icon of a **norepinephrine and dopamine** reuptake inhibitor (**NDRI**). In this case, four of the five pharmacological properties of the tricyclic antidepressants (TCAs) (Fig. 2–27) were removed. Only the norepinephrine reuptake inhibitor (**NRI**) portion remains; to this is added a dopamine reuptake inhibitor action (**DRI**).

1555U88 and tomoxetine, although Org4428 was dropped from further clinical development.

Norepinephrine and Dopamine Reuptake Blockers

Bupropion is the prototypical agent of the norepinephrine and dopamine reuptake inhibitors (Fig. 2–48). For many years, its mechanism of action was unclear. Bupropion itself has weak reuptake properties for dopamine, and weaker yet reuptake properties for norepinephrine. The action of the drug on norepinephrine and dopamine neurotransmission, however, has always appeared to be more powerful than these weak properties could explain, which has led to proposals that bupropion acts rather vaguely as an adrenergic modulator of some type. Bupropion is metabolized to an active metabolite, which is not only a more powerful norepinephrine reuptake blocker than bupropion itself but is also concentrated in the brain. In some ways, therefore, bupropion is more of a pro-drug (i.e., precursor) than a drug itself. That is, it gives rise to the "real" drug, namely its hydroxylated active metabolite, and it is this metabolite that is the actual mediator of antidepressant efficacy via norepinephrine and dopamine reuptake blockade (Fig. 2–49).

A sustained release formulation of bupropion (bupropion SR) has largely replaced immediate-release bupropion, not only because dosing frequency is reduced to only twice daily but also because of increased tolerability, especially an apparent reduction in the frequency of seizures associated with the immediate-release formulation.

Bupropion SR is generally activating or even stimulating. Interestingly, bupropion SR does not appear to be associated with production of the bothersome sexual dysfunction that can occur with the SSRIs, probably because bupropion lacks a significant serotonergic component to its mechanism of action. Thus, it may be a useful antidepressant not only for patients who cannot tolerate the serotonergic side effects of SSRIs, but also for patients whose depression does not respond to boosting

NDRI ACTION

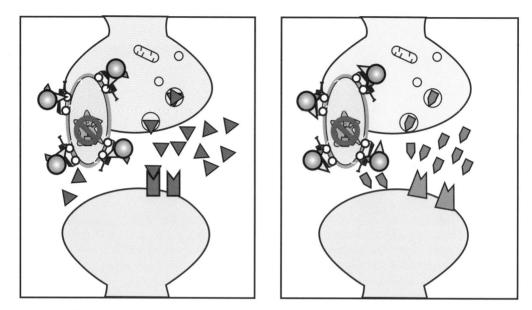

FIGURE 2–49. In this diagram, the norepinephrine reuptake inhibitor (**NRI**) and the dopamine reuptake inhibitor (**DRI**) portions of the **NDRI** molecule are shown inserted in the norepinephrine and the dopamine reuptake pumps, respectively, blocking them and causing an **antidepressant effect**.

serotonin by SSRIs. Bupropion SR is also useful in decreasing the craving associated with smoking cessation.

Other prodopaminergic agents are available as antidepressants in some countries, for example, amineptine in France and Brazil. Brasofensine, a dopamine reuptake blocker, is in clinical testing. Another vaguely prodopaminergic agent is modafinil, recently approved for the treatment of narcolepsy but not depression. It may act in part as a dopamine reuptake inhibitor but not a dopamine releaser like amphetamine. It may have theoretical antidepressant actions, but this has not been established in clinical trials. One potential worry that keeps pharmaceutical sponsors away from testing dopamine reuptake inhibitors as antidepressants is the possibility that they may be reinforcing and lead to abuse similar to stimulant abuse.

Summary

In this chapter, we have discussed the mechanisms of action of the major antidepressant drugs. The acute pharmacological actions of these agents on receptors and enzymes have been described, as well as the major hypothesis that attempts to explain how all current antidepressants ultimately work. That hypothesis is known as the neurotransmitter receptor hypothesis of antidepressant action. We have also introduced pharmacokinetic concepts relating to the metabolism of antidepressants and mood stabilizers by the cytochrome P450 enzyme system.

Specific antidepressant agents that the reader should now understand include the monoamine oxidase inhibitors, tricyclic antidepressants, serotonin selective reuptake inhibitors, and noradrenergic reuptake inhibitors, including both selective norepinephrine reuptake inhibitors and norepinephrine–dopamine reuptake inhibitors.

Although the specific pragmatic guidelines for use of these various therapeutic agents for depression have not been emphasized, the reader should now have a basis for the rational use of these antidepressant drugs founded on application of principles discussed earlier in this chapter, namely, drug actions on neurotransmission via actions at key receptors and enzymes. Other antidepressants and mood stabilizers, as well as how to combine them, are discussed in Chapter 3.

NEWER ANTIDEPRESSANTS AND MOOD STABILIZERS

In this chapter, we will continue our review of pharmacological concepts underlying the use of antidepressant and mood-stabilizing drugs. The goal of this chapter is to acquaint the reader with current ideas about how several of the newer antidepressants work. We will also introduce ideas about the pharmacologic mechanism of action of the mood stabilizers. As in Chapter 2, we will explain the mechanisms of action of these drugs by building on general pharmacological concepts.

Our treatment of antidepressants in this chapter continues at the conceptual level, and not at the pragmatic level. The reader should consult standard drug handbooks for details of doses, side effects, drug interactions, and other issues relevant to the prescribing of these drugs in clinical practice.

Discussion of antidepressants and mood stabilizers will begin with the antidepressants that act by a dual pharmacological mechanism, including dual reuptake blockade, alpha 2 antagonism and dual serotonin 2A antagonism/serotonin reuptake blockade. We will also explore several antidepressants under development but not

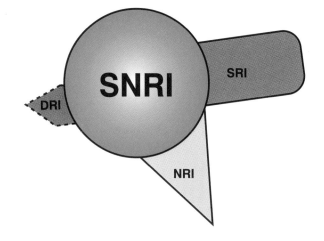

The **Serotonin-Norepinephrine reuptake inhibitor**
blocks the reuptake of norepinephrine and of serotonin.

FIGURE 3–1. Shown here is the icon of a dual reuptake inhibitor, which combines the actions of both a **serotonin** reuptake inhibitor (**SRI**) and a **norepinephrine** reuptake inhibitor (**NRI**). In this case, three of the five pharmacological properties of the tricyclic antidepressants (TCAs) (Fig. 2–27) were removed. Both the SRI portion and the NRI portion of the TCA remain; however the alpha, antihistamine, and anticholinergic portions are removed. These **serotonin/norepinephrine reuptake inhibitors** are called **SNRIs** or **dual inhibitors**. A small amount of dopamine reuptake inhibition (DRI) is also present in some of these agents, especially at high doses.

yet introduced into clinical practice. Next, we will introduce the use of lithium and anticonvulsants as mood stabilizers. Finally, we will discuss the use of combinations of drugs and briefly mention electroconvulsive therapy (ECT) and psychotherapy for the treatment of mood disorders.

Dual Serotonin and Norepinephrine Reuptake Inhibitors

One class of antidepressants that combines the actions of both the selective serotonin reuptake inhibitors (SSRIs) and the selective noreadrenergic reuptake inhibitors (NRIs) is the class of dual serotonin and noreadrenergic reuptake inhibitors (SNRIs) (Fig. 3–1). The designation "dual reuptake inhibitors" can be confusing because many tricyclic antidepressants (TCAs) are also dual reuptake inhibitors of both norepinephrine (NE) and serotonin (5-hydroxytryptamine {5HT}). What is unique about venlafaxine, the prototypical SNRI, is that it shares the NE and 5HT, and to a lesser extent dopamine (DA) reuptake inhibitory properties of the classical TCAs (Fig. 3–1), but without alpha 1, cholinergic, or histamine receptor blocking properties (see Figs. 2–30 to 2–32). Thus, SNRIs are not only dual-action agents, but they are **selective** for this dual action. Dual-action SNRIs thus have the properties of an SSRI and a selective NRI added together in the same molecule.

Venlafaxine is the only dual-action SNRI currently marketed. Depending on the dose, it has different degrees of inhibition of 5HT reuptake (most potent and therefore present at low doses), NE reuptake (moderate potency and therefore present at higher doses) and DA reuptake (least potent and therefore present only at highest doses) (Fig. 3–2). However, there are no significant actions on other receptors. Venlafaxine is now available in an extended-release formulation (venlafaxine XR), which not only allows once daily administration but also significantly reduces side effects, especially nausea. The increased tolerability of venlafaxine in this new formulation is important, especially considering the trend in psychiatry to use higher doses of venlafaxine XR to exploit both the NE and the 5HT mechanism.

Additional dual 5HT-NE reuptake inhibitors include sibutramine, which is approved for the treatment of obesity but not depression. Tramadol is a kappa opiate agonist approved for the treatment of pain, but it also has serotonin and norepinephrine reuptake inhibitor properties. Dual reuptake inhibitors in clinical testing as antidepressants include milnacipran and duloxetine.

Are two antidepressant mechanisms better than one? The original tricyclic antidepressants have multiple pharmacological mechanisms and are termed "dirty drugs" because many of these mechanisms were undesirable, as they cause side effects (Fig. 3–3). The idea was then to "clean up" these agents by making them selective, and thus the SSRI era was born. Indeed, developing such selective agents made them devoid of pharmacologic properties that mediated anticholinergic, antihistaminic, and antiadrenergic side effects (Fig. 3–3). However, selectivity may sometimes be less desired than multiple pharmacologic mechanisms, as in difficult cases that are

SNRI ACTIONS

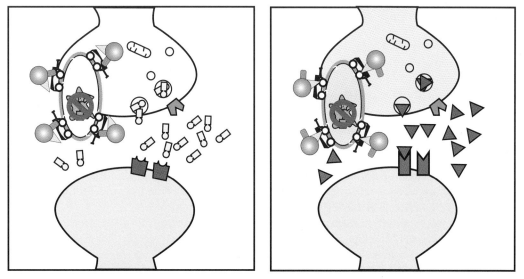

FIGURE 3–2. In this diagram, the dual actions of the serotonin/norepinephrine reuptake inhibitors (**SNRIs**) are shown. Both the norepinephrine reuptake inhibitor (NRI) portion of the SNRI molecule (left panel) and the serotonin reuptake inhibitor (SRI) portion of the SNRI molecule are inserted into their respective reuptake pumps. Consequently, both reuptake pumps are blocked, and the drug mediates an **antidepressant effect**. This is analogous to two of the dimensions of the tricyclic antidepressants (TCAs), already shown in Figures 2–28 and 2–29. It is also analogous to the single action of SSRIs (Fig. 2–33) added to the single action of the selective NRIs (Figure 2–46).

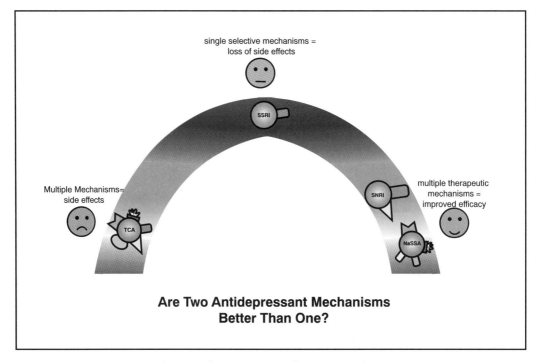

**Are Two Antidepressant Mechanisms
Better Than One?**

FIGURE 3–3. Are **two mechanisms** better than one for some antidepressants? Originally, multiple mechanisms were synonymous with "dirty drugs" because they implied unwanted side effects. This is shown as tricyclic antidepressants on the left. The trend to develop selective drugs (center) led to removal of unwanted side effects. More recently, the trend has again been to add multiple mechanisms together to improve tolerability and enhance efficacy. **Enhanced efficacy** from synergistic pharmacological mechanisms can apparently increase therapeutic responses in some patients, especially those resistant to single-mechanism agents.

resistant to treatment with drugs having a selective serotonergic mechanism. Thus, more recently psychotropic drug development has been trending back to multiple pharmacologic mechanisms in the hope that this would exploit potential synergies among two or more independent therapeutic mechanisms. For antidepressants, this has led to the development of drugs that exhibit "intramolecular polypharmacy," such as the dual SNRIs discussed here (Fig. 3–3). It has also led to the increasing use of two antidepressants together for treatment-resistant cases, combining two or more synergistic therapeutic mechanisms, as discussed below.

Thus, not only are dual-reuptake inhibitors effective antidepressants, but they may have some therapeutic advantages over the SSRIs. Theoretically, the addition of NE, and to a lesser extent DA, reuptake blockade to 5HT reuptake blockade (Fig. 3–2) might lead to pharmacological synergy among these neurotransmitter systems and thus boost efficacy. Synergy is the working together of two or more mechanisms so that the total efficacy is greater than the sum of its parts (in other words, 1 + 1 = 10).

The molecular basis of this synergy may be manifest at the level of genetic expression. Thus, beta-adrenergic receptor stimulation by NE results in gene expression, as discussed previously and shown in Figure 3–4. However, in the presence of

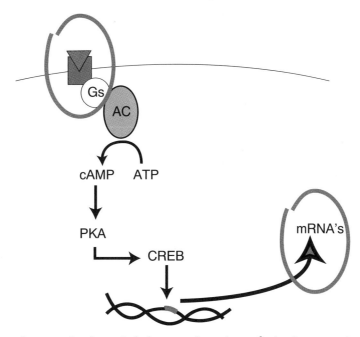

FIGURE 3–4. Shown here are the theoretical **therapeutic actions** of selective serotonin antidepressants on **gene expression**. The purple norepinephrine (NE) at the top (top red circle) is causing a cascade of biochemical events resulting in the transcription of a neuron's genes (mRNAs in the bottom circle). The noradrenergic receptor is linked to a stimulatory G protein (Gs), which is linked in turn to the enzyme adenylate cyclase (AC), which converts ATP into the second messenger cAMP. Next, cAMP activates protein kinase A (PKA), which then activates a transcription factor such as cyclic AMP response element binding (CREB) protein.

simultaneous serotonin 2A receptor stimulation by serotonin, gene expression is amplified synergistically (Fig. 3–5). Thus, norepinephrine and serotonin may work together to produce critical expression of genes in a manner that does not occur when either works alone. This could theoretically explain why dual 5HT-NE reuptake blockade may produce synergistic antidepressant effects in some patients.

Indications that there may be antidepressant synergy from dual 5HT-NE actions that correspond with these theoretical molecular events comes from studies in which venlafaxine has produced increased remission rates in major depressive disorders as compared with SSRIs. Increased remission rates with the TCAs over the SSRIs have also been reported and support the concept of dual action being more efficacious than SSRI action alone for remission of depression in some patients.

Another indication that the dual mechanisms may lead to more efficacy is the finding that venlafaxine seems to have greater efficacy as the dose increases, whereas other antidepressants seem to have little difference in efficacy at higher doses. Since the noradrenergic (and dopaminergic) action of venlafaxine is greater at higher doses, this suggests that there is more and more efficacy as the second mechanism becomes active (i.e., the noradrenergic "boost"). This also supports the rationale for using dual mechanisms for the most difficult patients, (i.e., those who are treatment-resistant to SSRIs and other antidepressants and those who are responders but not remitters to SSRIs or other antidepressants).

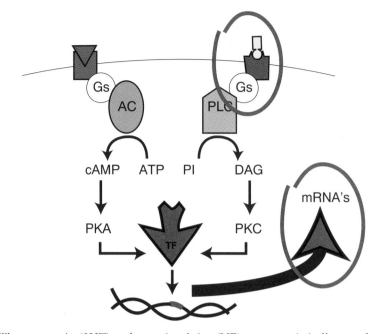

FIGURE 3–5. When serotonin (5HT) and norepinephrine (NE) act synergistically to **enhance gene expression** (compare with Fig. 3–4), this theoretically results in enhanced therapeutic efficacy in depression. Thus, the cascade on the left (shown also in Fig. 3–4) here is occurring simultaneously with the activation of the cascade on the right. Serotonin (top red circle) is thus working with NE on the left to cause even more gene activation (mRNAs in the bottom red circle) than NE can cause by itself in Figure 3–4. This is **synergy**. The 5HT receptor here is coupled to a stimulatory G protein (Gs), which activates the enzyme phospholipase C (PLC) to convert phosphatidyl inositol (PI) to diacylglycerol (DAG) and activate calcium flux, so that protein kinase C (PKC) can increase the transcription of neuronal genes by working synergistically at the level of transcription factors (TF).

Other information suggesting therapeutic advantages for dual mechanisms is the finding that the SNRI venlafaxine XR is an effective generalized anxiolytic. That is, among the known antidepressants only venlafaxine XR is approved as a generalized anxiolytic as well as an antidepressant. Such actions might have the favorable therapeutic consequences of converting anxious depression into complete remission of *both* depression and anxiety. Additional support for the role of dual SNRI action yielding enhanced efficacy in both depression and anxiety comes from evidence that the dual-action but nonselective tricyclic antidepressants also appear to be effective as generalized anxiolytics but have never been marketed for this indication. Dual-action mirtazapine may also have some generalized anxiolytic effects (see below).

There are a number of ways to implement this dual mechanism strategy beyond just using higher doses of venlafaxine XR. One of these is to use other dual 5HT/NE–acting antidepressants, such as mirtazapine, discussed below, or possibly even going back to certain tricyclic antidepressants or monoamine oxidase inhibitors (MAOIs). Another would be to use pharmacologically rational combinations of drugs with potentially synergistic mechanisms. An obvious example of how to deliver dual serotonin and noradrenergic reuptake inhibition would be to add reboxetine to an SSRI. This and other dual mechanism strategies will be discussed in further detail in the section on antidepressant combinations.

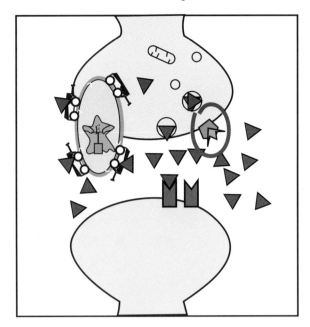

FIGURE 3–6. **Alpha 2 antagonists** (red circle) can increase noradrenergic neurotransmission by "cutting the brake cable" for noradrenergic neurons. That is, alpha 2 antagonists block presynaptic alpha 2 autoreceptors (red circle), which are the "brakes" on noradrenergic neurons. This causes noradrenergic neurons to become disinhibited, since norepinephrine (NE) can no longer block its own release. Thus, **noradrenergic** neurotransmission is **enhanced**.

Dual Serotonin and Norepinephrine Actions Via Alpha 2 Antagonism

Blocking the reuptake pump for monoamines or the enzyme monoamine oxidase (MAO) are not the only mechanisms to increase serotonin and norepinephrine. Another way to raise both serotonin and norepinephrine levels is to block alpha 2 receptors. Recall that norepinephrine turns off its own release by interacting with presynaptic alpha 2 autoreceptors on noreadrenergic neurons (Fig. 1–21); norepinephrine also turns off serotonin release by interacting with presynaptic alpha 2 heteroreceptors on serotonergic neurons (Fig. 1–44). If an alpha 2 antagonist is administered, norepinephrine can no longer turn off its own release, and noradrenergic neurons are thus disinhibited (Fig. 3–6). That is, the alpha 2 antagonist "cuts the brake cable" of the noradrenergic neuron, and norepinephrine release is thereby increased.

Similarly, alpha 2 antagonists do not allow norepinephrine to turn off serotonin release. Therefore, serotonergic neurons become disinhibited (Fig. 3–7). Similarly to their actions at noradrenergic neurons, alpha 2 antagonists act at serotonergic neurons to "cut the brake cable" of noradrenergic inhibition norepinephrine brake on serotonin shown in Figs. 1–47 and 1–48. Serotonin release is therefore increased (Fig. 3–7).

A second mechanism to increase serotonin release after administration of an alpha 2 antagonist may be even more important. Recall that norepinephrine neurons from the locus coeruleus innervate the cell bodies of serotonergic neurons in the midbrain raphe (Figs. 1–47 and 1–48). This noradrenergic input enhances serotonin release

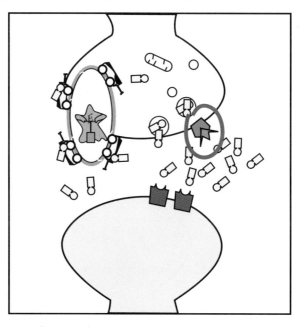

FIGURE 3–7. **Alpha 2 antagonists** can also increase serotonergic neurotransmission by "cutting the brake cable" for serotonergic neurons (compare with Fig. 3–6). That is, alpha 2 antagonists block presynaptic alpha 2 heteroreceptors (red circle), the "brakes" on serotonergic neurons. This causes serotonergic neurons to become disinhibited, since norepinephrine (NE) can no longer block serotonin (5HT) release. Thus, **serotonergic** neurotransmission is **enhanced**.

via a postsynaptic alpha 1 receptor. Thus, when norepinephrine is disinhibited in the noradrenergic pathway to the raphe, the norepinephrine release there will increase and cause alpha 1 receptors to be stimulated, thereby provoking more serotonin release (Fig. 3–8). This is like stepping on the serotonin accelerator. Thus, alpha 2 antagonists both cut the brake cable and step on the accelerator for serotonin release (Fig. 3–9).

Alpha 2 antagonist actions thus yield dual enhancement of both serotonin and norepinephrine release (Fig. 3–10). Although no selective alpha 2 antagonist is available for use as an antidepressant, one drug with prominent alpha 2 properties, namely mirtazapine, is available worldwide as an antidepressant (Fig. 3–10). Mirtazapine does not block any monoamine transporter, but in addition to its potent antagonist actions on alpha 2 receptors it also has antagonist actions at serotonin 2A, 2C, and 3 receptors and histamine 1 receptors (Fig. 3–10). The 5HT2A antagonist properties may contribute to mirtazapine's antidepressant actions (Fig. 3–11), and these serotonin 2A antagonist properties as well as serotonin 2C antagonist and H1 antihistamine properties may contribute to its anxiolytic and sedative hypnotic properties (Figs. 3–11 to 3–13). By blocking serotonin 2A, 2C, and 3 receptors, the side effects associated with stimulating them, especially anxiety, nausea, and sexual dysfunction are avoided (Fig. 3–11). However, blocking serotonin 2A and H1 antihistamine receptors accounts for the side effect of sedation, and blocking serotonin 2C and H1 receptors accounts for the side effect of weight gain (Fig. 3–12).

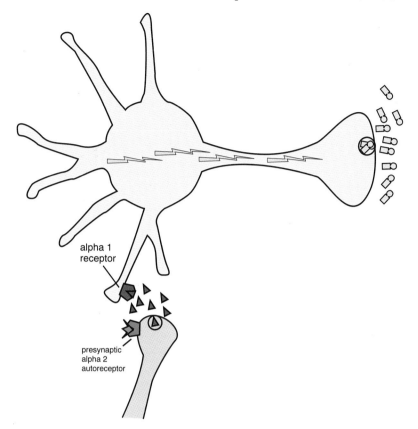

FIGURE 3–8. **Alpha 2 antagonists** can also **increase serotonergic neurotransmission** by "stepping on the serotonin (5HT) accelerator." That is, norepinephrine (NE) input for the locus coeruleus (bottom) to the cell bodies of serotonergic neurons in the midbrain raphe synapse on postsynaptic excitatory alpha 1 receptors. This **increases** serotonergic neuronal firing and serotonin release from the serotonin nerve terminal on the right.

The therapeutic actions of mirtazapine are thought to be mainly mediated through its alpha 2 antagonist properties. As mentioned above, by blocking presynaptic alpha 2 receptors, mirtazapine cuts the brake cable and disinhibits both serotonin and norepinephrine release; by disinhibiting norepinephrine release, alpha 1 receptors are stimulated by norepinephrine, and serotonin release is enhanced by stepping on the serotonin accelerator (Fig. 3–13). An integrated view of all of mirtazapine's pharmacologic actions is shown in Figure 3–13.

In addition to its efficacy as a first-line antidepressant, mirtazapine may have enhanced efficacy due to its dual mechanism of action (Fig. 3–3), especially in combination with other antidepressants that block serotonin and/or norepinephrine reuptake. This will be discussed below in the section on antidepressant combinations. Mirtazapine may also have utility in panic disorder, generalized anxiety disorder, and other anxiety disorders, but has not been intensively studied for these indications.

Two other alpha 2 antagonists are marketed as antidepressants in some countries (but not the United States), namely, mianserin (worldwide except in the United

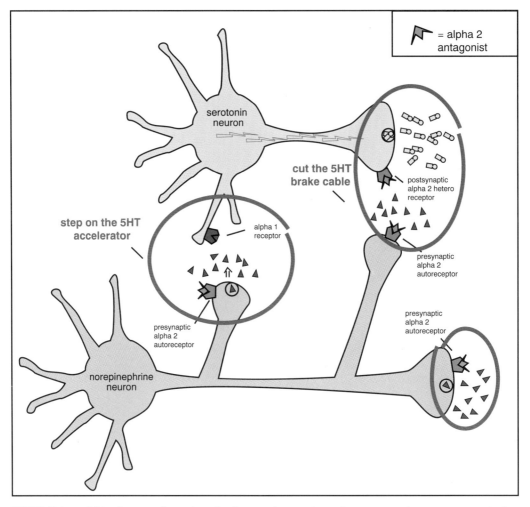

FIGURE 3–9. This diagram shows how **both noradrenergic and serotonergic neurotransmission are enhanced by alpha 2 antagonists.** The noradrenergic neuron at the bottom is interacting with the serotonergic neuron at the top. The noradrenergic neuron is disinhibited at all of its axon terminals because an alpha 2 antagonist is blocking all of its presynaptic alpha 2 autoreceptors. Thus, this has the effect of "cutting the brake cables" for norepinephrine (NE) release at all of its noradrenergic nerve terminals (NE released in all three red circles). Serotonin (5HT) release is enhanced by NE via two distinct mechanisms. First, alpha 2 antagonists "step on the 5HT accelerator" when NE stimulates alpha 1 receptors on the 5HT cell body and dendrites (left red circle). Second, alpha 2 antagonists "cut the 5HT brake cable" when alpha 2 presynaptic heteroreceptors are blocked on the 5HT axon terminal (middle red circle).

States) and setiptilene (Japan). Mianserin has alpha 1 antagonist properties, which mitigate the effects of enhancing serotonergic neurotransmission, so that this drug enhances predominantly noradrenergic neurotransmission, yet with associated 5HT2A, 5HT2C, 5HT3, and H1 antagonist properties. Yohimbine is also an alpha 2 antagonist, but its alpha 1 antagonist properties similarly mitigate its pro-monoaminergic actions. Several selective alpha 2 antagonists, including idazoxan and fluparoxan, have been tested, but they have not yet demonstrated robust antide-

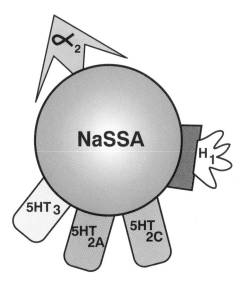

FIGURE 3–10. Icon for **mirtazapine**, sometimes also called a noradrenergic and specific serotonergic antidepressant (NaSSA). Its primary therapeutic action is alpha 2 antagonism as shown in Figures 3–6 through 3–9. It also blocks three serotonin receptors: 5HT2A, 5HT2C, and 5HT3. Finally, it blocks H1 histamine receptors.

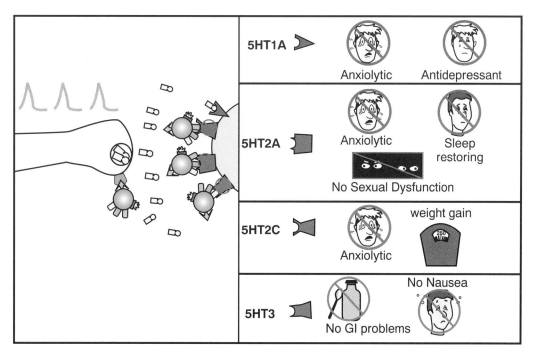

FIGURE 3–11. **Mirtazapine** actions at **serotonin** (5HT) synapses. When presynaptic alpha 2 heteroreceptors are blocked, 5HT is released, but it is directed to the 5HT1A receptor because 5HT actions at 5HT2A, 5HT2C, and 5HT3 receptors are blocked. The result is that antidepressant and anxiolytic actions are preserved but the side effects associated with stimulating 5HT2A, 5HT2C, and 5HT3 receptors are blocked. However, sedation and weight gain may result from these actions.

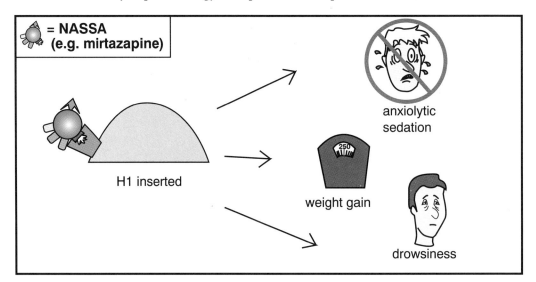

FIGURE 3–12. When **mirtazapine** blocks **histamine** 1 receptors, it can cause anxiolytic actions, but also sedation and weight gain as side effects.

pressant efficacy and also are not always well tolerated because they can provoke panic, anxiety, and prolonged erections in men.

Dual Serotonin 2 Antagonists/Serotonin Reuptake Inhibitors

Several antidepressants share the ability to block serotonin 2A receptors as well as serotonin reuptake. In fact, some of the tricyclic antidepressants, such as amitriptyline, nortriptyline, doxepin, and especially amoxapine, have this combination of actions at the serotonin synapse. Since the potency of blockade of serotonin 2A receptors varies considerably among the tricyclics, it is not clear how important this action is to the therapeutic actions of tricyclic antidepressants in general.

However, there is another chemical class of antidepressants known as phenylpiperazines, which are more selective than the tricyclic antidepressants and whose most powerful pharmacological action is to block serotonin 2A receptors (Fig. 3–14). This includes the agents nefazodone and trazodone. Both of these agents also block serotonin reuptake but do so in a less potent manner than either the tricyclic antidepressants or the SSRIs (Fig. 3–15). Since the pharmacological mechanism of action of dual serotonin 2A antagonist/serotonin reuptake inhibitors derives from a combination of powerful antagonism of serotonin 2A receptors with less powerful blockade of serotonin reuptake, these agents are classified separately as serotonin 2A antagonists/reuptake inhibitors (*SARIs*) (Figs. 3–14 and 3–15).

Nefazodone is the prototypical member of the SARI class of antidepressants. It is a powerful serotonin 2A antagonist with secondary actions as a serotonin and norepinephrine reuptake inhibitor (Figs. 3–14 and 3–15). Nefazodone also blocks alpha 1 receptors, but the clinical consequences of this are generally not important, perhaps because its norepinephrine reuptake inhibition reduces this action *in vivo*.

The major distinction between the SARIs and other classes of antidepressants is that SARIs are predominantly 5HT2A antagonists. A lesser but important amount

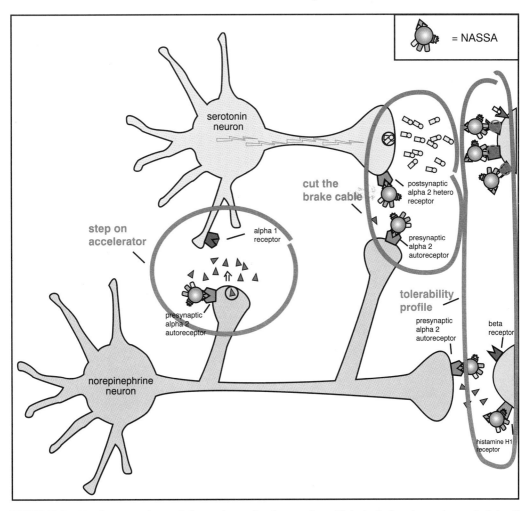

= NASSA

serotonin
neuron

cut the
brake cable

postsynaptic
alpha 2 hetero
receptor

step on
accelerator

alpha 1
receptor

presynaptic
alpha 2
autoreceptor

tolerability
profile

presynaptic
alpha 2
autoreceptor

presynaptic
alpha 2
autoreceptor

beta
receptor

norepinephrine
neuron

histamine H1
receptor

FIGURE 3–13. An **overview** of the actions of **mirtazapine**. This includes the actions of alpha 2 antagonists already shown in Figure 3–9, that is, the therapeutic actions of cutting the NE brake cable while stepping on the 5HT accelerator (left circle), as well as cutting the 5HT brake cable (middle circle). This increases both 5HT and NE neurotransmission. On the right are the additional actions of mirtazapine beyond alpha 2 antagonism. These postsynaptic actions mainly account for the tolerability profile of mirtazapine.

of 5HT reuptake inhibition also occurs. That is, the SARI nefazodone may exploit the natural antagonism between 5HT1A and 5HT2A receptors by increasing 5HT through reuptake blockade while simultaneously blocking its actions at 5HT2A receptors. Normally, stimulation of 5HT2A receptors mitigates the stimulation of 5HT1A receptors (Figs. 3–16 and 3–17). This may also play out at the level of gene expression, where gene expression by 5HT1A stimulation alone (Fig. 3–18) is opposed by simultaneous stimulation of 5HT2A receptors (Fig. 3–19).

On the other hand, if 5HT2A receptors are blocked rather than stimulated, the normal inhibiting influence on 5HT1A receptor stimulation is lost. This may indirectly boost the effects of stimulating 5HT1A receptors, since it is no longer

Serotonin Antagonist/Reuptake Inhibitors (SARIs)

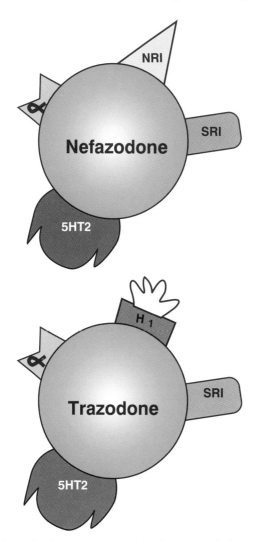

FIGURE 3–14. Shown here are icons for two of the serotonin 2A antagonist/reuptake inhibitors (SARIs). Nefazodone is the prototype agent in this class, which also includes trazodone. These agents also have a **dual action**, but the two mechanisms are different from the dual actions of the serotonin norepinephrine reuptake inhibitors (SNRIs). The SARIs act by potent **blockade of serotonin 2A (5HT2A) receptors, combined with less potent serotonin reuptake inhibitor (SRI) actions**. Nefazodone also has weak norepinephrine reuptake inhibition (NRI) as well as weak alpha 1 adrenergic blocking properties. Trazodone also contains antihistamine properties and alpha 1 antagonist properties but lacks the NRI properties of nefazodone.

124

SARI (NEFAZODONE) ACTIONS AT 5HT SYNAPSES

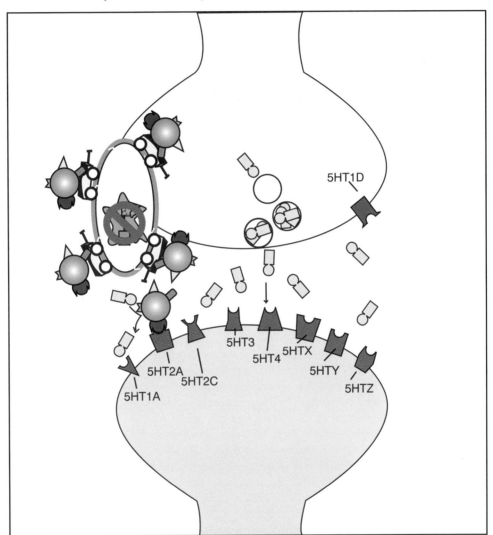

FIGURE 3–15. This diagram shows the dual actions of the **serotonin 2A antagonist/reuptake inhibitor (SARI) nefazodone**. This agent acts both presynaptically and postsynaptically. Presynaptic actions are indicated by the serotonin reuptake inhibitor (**SRI**) portion of the icon, which is inserted into the serotonin reuptake pump, blocking it. Postsynaptic actions are indicated by the **serotonin 2A receptor antagonist** portion of the icon (5HT2A), inserted into the serotonin 2 receptor, blocking it. It is believed that both actions contribute to the antidepressant actions of nefazodone. Blocking serotonin actions at 5HT2A receptors may also diminish side effects mediated by stimulation of 5HT2A receptors when the SRI acts to increase 5HT at all receptor subtypes. The serotonin 2A antagonist properties are stronger than the serotonin reuptake properties, so serotonin antagonism predominates at the 5HT2A receptor.

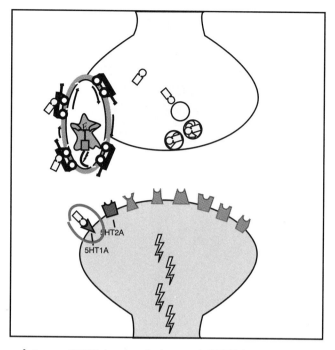

FIGURE 3–16. *Synergy between 5HT1A stimulation and 5HT2A antagonism*–part 1. Shown here is the pharmacologic action of 5HT1A stimulation alone (red circle).

mitigated by 5HT2A stimulation (Fig. 3–20). This same phenomenon may occur at the gene level as well (Fig. 3–21).

The SARI nefazodone may therefore not mediate its therapeutic actions merely by blocking 5HT2A receptors. In fact, selective 5HT2A antagonists have been tested in depression and have not been shown to be particularly efficacious antidepressants. The action of increasing 5HT via reuptake inhibition, leading to stimulation of 5HT1A receptors, may therefore be an important part of nefazodone's action. Without 5HT1A stimulation, 5HT2A antagonism would have nothing to potentiate. This principle will be discussed in further detail in the section on antidepressant combinations in which SSRIs are combined with other 5HT2A antagonists such as the atypical antipsychotics for resistant cases of depression. Combining indirect 5HT1A agonism with direct 5HT2A antagonism is another example of "intramolecular polypharmacy," exploiting the synergy that exists between these two mechanisms and again suggesting that two antidepressant mechanisms may sometimes be better than one.

When 5HT reuptake is inhibited selectively, as with the SSRIs, it causes essentially all serotonin receptors to be stimulated by the increased levels of 5HT that result. Although this has proved to be quite useful for treating depression and other disorders, it also has its costs. For example, we have discussed how stimulation of 5HT1A receptors in the raphe may help depression (Fig. 1–52), but how stimulating 5HT2A and 5HT2C receptors in the limbic cortex may cause agitation or anxiety (Figs. 1–53 and 1–54), and how stimulating 5HT2A receptors in the spinal cord may lead to sexual dysfunction (Fig. 1–57). Thus, an agent that combines 5HT

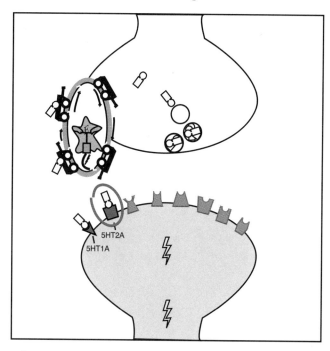

FIGURE 3–17. *Synergy between 5HT1A stimulation and 5HT2A antagonism*–part 2. Stimulation of 5HT2A receptors by 5HT (red circle) reduces the actions of 5HT at 5HT1A receptors (compare with Fig. 3–16).

reuptake blockade with stronger 5HT2A antagonism would theoretically reduce the undesired actions of 5HT when it stimulates 5HT2A receptors. In this case, competition between 5HT reuptake blockade and stronger 5HT2A antagonism results in net antagonism at the 5HT2A receptor. In fact, the SARI nefazodone thus theoretically lacks the potential to cause sexual dysfunction, and usually also insomnia and anxiety, associated with the SSRIs.

Clinical experience suggests that nefazodone may also be useful in panic disorder, posttraumatic stress disorder, and generalized anxiety disorder, but without the 5HT2A-activating side effects associated with the SSRIs.

Trazodone is the original member of the SARI group of antidepresssants. It also blocks alpha 1 receptors and histamine receptors (Fig. 3–14). Perhaps because of its histamine receptor blocking properties, it is extremely sedating. For this reason, its antidepressant use tends to be limited, yet it is well accepted as an excellent non-dependence-forming hypnotic, but it was never actually marketed for this indication. Its sedative hypnotic doses are generally lower than its effective antidepressant doses. Trazodone is used mostly as an adjunct to antidepressants because it not only increases the tolerability of SSRIs by blocking their side effects associated with stimulating 5HT2A receptors, such as insomnia and agitation, but it also can enhance the therapeutic efficacy of SSRIs, perhaps by exploiting the synergy of blocking 5HT2A receptors while stimulating 5HT1A receptors as discussed above. A rare but troublesome side effect of trazodone is priapism (prolonged erections in men, usually painful), which is treated by injecting alpha adrenergic agonists into the penis to reverse the priapism and prevent vascular damage to the penis.

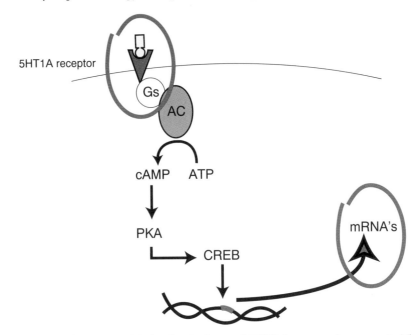

FIGURE 3–18. *Synergy between 5HT1A stimulation and 5HT2A antagonism*–part 3. The molecular consequences of 5HT1A stimulation alone, shown here, result in a certain amount of gene
expression corresponding to the pharmacological actions shown in Figure 3–16. Serotonin (5HT)
occupancy of its 5HT1A receptor (top red circle) causes a certain amount of gene transcription (see
bottom red circle on the right). The 5HT1A receptor is coupled to a stimulatory G protein (Gs) and
adenylate cyclase (AC), which produces the second messenger cyclic AMP from ATP. This in turn
activates protein kinase A (PKA), so that transcription factors such as cyclic AMP response element
binding protein (CREB) can activate gene expression (mRNAs).

Nefazodone is in clinical testing as an extended-release formulation, which will
reduce its administration to once daily and may also reduce its side effects. YM992
is another serotonin 2A antagonist with serotonin reuptake inhibition properties
that is in testing as an antidepressant. Other more selective 5HT2 antagonists have
been tested and discarded as potential antidepressants, including ritanserin and ame-
sergide. However, MDL-100907 and SR46349 are selective 5HT2A antagonists in
testing for schizophrenia. Furthermore, drugs with serotonin 2A antagonist properties but also dopamine antagonist properties, called serotonin-dopamine antagonists, or atypical antipsychotics, are in testing for bipolar disorder and for treatment-
resistant depression. They will be discussed in further detail in the sections of this
chapter below on bipolar disorder/antidepressant combinations. Agents with 5HT2A
antagonist properties but also 5HT1A agonist properties are in testing as potential
novel antidepressants; these include flibanserin, and possibly adatanserin and
BMS181,101.

New Antidepressants in Development

Currently, what is needed is an antidepressant that has onset of action faster than 2
to 8 weeks and has efficacy in more than two out of three patients. That efficacy

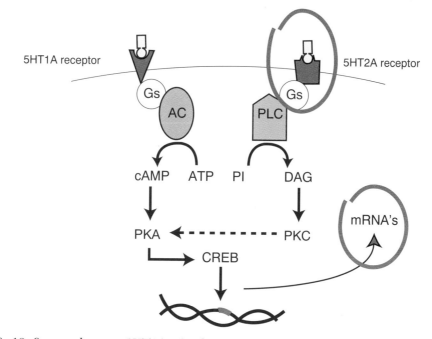

FIGURE 3–19. *Synergy between 5HT1A stimulation and 5HT2A antagonism*–part 4. The molecular consequences of 5HT2A receptor stimulation concomitant with 5HT1A receptor stimulation is to reduce the gene expression of 5HT1A stimulation alone (i.e., that shown in Fig. 3–18). These molecular consequences correlate with the pharmacologic actions of simultaneous 5HT1A and 5HT2A stimulation shown in Figure 3–17. Simultaneous activation of the 5HT2A receptor by serotonin (on the right) will alter the consequences of activating 5HT1A receptors in a negative way and reduce the gene expression of 5HT1A receptors acting alone (Fig. 3–18). Thus, occupancy of the 5HT2A receptor (top circle) causes coupling of a stimulatory G protein (Gs) with the enzyme phospholipase C (PLC). This, in turn, activates calcium flux and converts phosphatidylinositol (PI) into diacylglycerol (DAG). This activates the enzyme phosphokinase C (PKC), which has an inhibitory action on phosphokinase A (PKA). This reduces the activation of transcription factors such as cyclic AMP response element binding protein (CREB) and leads to a decrease in gene expression (bottom red circle).

should be robust, causing remission, not response, and sustaining that remission for longer periods of time and in a larger proportion of patients than current antidepressants. Several theoretical candidates are in development, and some related to the mechanisms discussed above have already been mentioned. A sampling of other potential candidate antidepressants is given below. Most are variations on the theme of modulating either adrenergic neurons or serotonergic neurons with novel pharmacological mechanisms. Others attempt to achieve antidepressant actions by modulating peptide systems.

Monoaminergic Modulators

Beta agonists. Beta adrenergic receptors can be rapidly down regulated by agonists and if this is desired for an antidepressant action, beta agonists may be useful. To date, it has not been possible to identify beta 1 or beta 2 agonists that successfully penetrate the brain and yet are not cardiotoxic. Pursuing safer beta 1 and beta 2

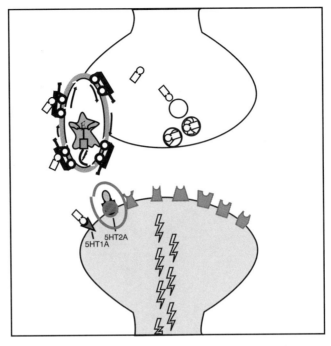

FIGURE 3–20. *Synergy between 5HT1A stimulation and 5HT2A antagonism*–part 5. If 5HT2A receptors are pharmacologically blocked rather than stimulated, they can no longer inhibit 5HT1A actions. Thus, 5HT1A receptors are disinhibited (compare with Figs. 3–16 and 3–17).

agonists, perhaps as partial agonists, may optimize the pharmacological properties. However, beta 3 agonists such as SR58611 show preclinical efficacy as antidepressants and are in preliminary clinical testing.

Second messenger systems. Enhancing adrenergic functioning distal to the receptor occupancy site can theoretically be accomplished by targeting either the G proteins or the adenylate cyclase enzyme. Both types of agents are under development. Rolipram has shown promise in the past as an antidepressant that blocks the destruction of cyclic adenosine monophospate (cAMP) second messengers. Lithium mimetics that act on monoamine receptor G proteins or on enzymes regulating phosphatidyl inositol second messenger systems are being tested preclinically. It may turn out fortuitously that some of the anticonvulsants known or suspected to be useful for bipolar disorder, including depression, act on second messenger systems. Further exploitation of this approach may have to await clarification of the biochemical cascade that regulates critical gene expression in monoaminergic neurons and their targets.

5HT1A agonists, partial agonists and antagonists. Although many 5HT1A agonists have been extensively tested in clinical trials, none has made it to the market as an antidepressant, and only one has been approved as a generalized anxiolytic. Several 5HT1A agonists and partial agonists have been dropped from clinical development, but others still survive in clinical research. Gepirone ER, a chemical cousin of bus-

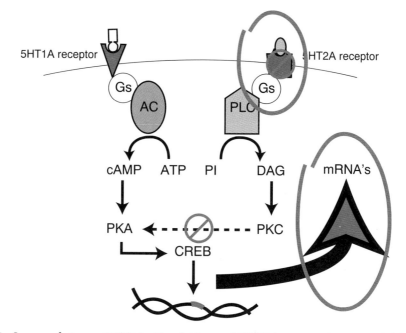

FIGURE 3−21. *Synergy between 5HT1A stimulation and 5HT2A antagonism*−part 6. The molecular consequences of 5HT1A receptor disinhibition by 5HT2A receptor blockade is shown here, namely enhanced gene expression. These molecular events are the consequence of the pharmacological actions shown in Figure 3−20. Simultaneous inhibition of the 5HT2A receptor on the right can stop the negative consequences that 5HT2A receptor stimulation by 5HT can have on gene expression, as shown in Figure 3−19. Thus, gene expression of the 5HT1A receptor (Fig. 3−18) is enhanced when 5HT2A receptors are blocked (bottom red circle) rather than diminished when they are stimulated (Fig. 3−19). The molecular basis of these effects is best reviewed by comparing Figures 3−18, 3−19, and 3−21. The pharmacological basis of these effects is best reviewed by comparing Figures 3−16, 3−17, and 3−20.

pirone, is continuing in clinical development in the United States and tandospirone in Japan. Ipsapirone, sunepitron, transdermal buspirone, and others have been dropped from clinical development, although there may be some continuing interest in flesinoxan or others.

Theoretically, a 5HT1A antagonist might be a rapid-onset antidepressant owing to immediate disinhibition of the serotonin neuron. This has been demonstrated preclinically, but no selective 5HT1A antagonist has undergone clinical testing in depression.

Serotonin and dopamine reuptake inhibition. Dual reuptake blockers of both serotonin and dopamine are in clinical testing. Although the SSRI sertraline has some dopamine reuptake inhibition as well as more potent serotonin reuptake inhibition, minaprine and bazinaprine have more potent dopamine actions and are thus dual serotonin/dopamine agents.

Serotonin 1D antagonists. Theoretically, a 5HT1A antagonist should rapidly disinhibit the serotonin neuron and be a rapid-onset antidepressant. One such compound CP-448,187 is entering clinical development.

Neurokinin Antagonists

As explained in Chapter 1, theoretical considerations and some serendipitous clinical observations suggest that neurokinin antagonists, especially NK1 antagonists (i.e., substance P antagonists) may be novel antidepressants. Thus clinical testing is underway on NK1 antagonists including SR140333, MK-869, L-760,735, L-733,060, CP-96,345, and CP-122,721, as well as several others; NK2 antagonists such as SR48968 and GR-159,897; and NK3 antagonists such as SR142801.

Novel Neurotransmitter Mechanisms

Other potentially novel antidepressants in clinical testing target different neurotransmitter systems, including sigma receptors, peptides such as neurotensin or cholecystokinin, and endogenous reward systems such as anandamide. These are in their very early testing phase.

Herbs

Herbal medicines such as hypericum, the active ingredient in St. John's wort, are used widely throughout the world, although never proven to be antidepressants by the same level of scrutiny as drugs marketed as antidepressants, such as TCAs and SSRIs. However, legitimate high-standard clinical testing is in progress to see whether herbs, especially St. John's wort, will prove to be antidepressants when held up to the same scrutiny that any drug undergoes prior to being marketed as an antidepressant. Recent reports that St. John's wort may have some toxic effect on reproductive functioning may mitigate the enthusiasm for this approach, however. One study suggests that it negatively affects fertility in both men and women. In addition, there is some evidence for mutation of the gene in sperm cells that may possibly increase risk to the developing fetus. Therefore, pregnancy is not currently recommended while taking these herbs.

Mood-Stabilizing Drugs

Lithium, the Classical Mood Stabilizer

Mood disorders characterized by elevations of mood above normal as well as depressions below normal are classically treated with lithium, an ion whose mechanism of action is not certain. Candidates for its mechanism of action are sites beyond the receptor in the second messenger system, perhaps either as an inhibitor of an enzyme, called inositol monophosphatase, involved in the phosphatidyl inositol system as a modulator of G proteins, or even as a regulator of gene expression by modulating protein kinase C (Fig. 3–22).

Lithium not only treats acute episodes of mania and hypomania but was the first psychotropic agent shown to prevent recurrent episodes of illness. Lithium may also be effective in treating and preventing episodes of depression in patients with bipolar disorder. It is least effective for rapid cycling or mixed episodes. Overall, lithium is effective in only 40 to 50% of patients. Furthermore, many patients are unable to tolerate it because of numerous side effects, including gastrointestinal symptoms

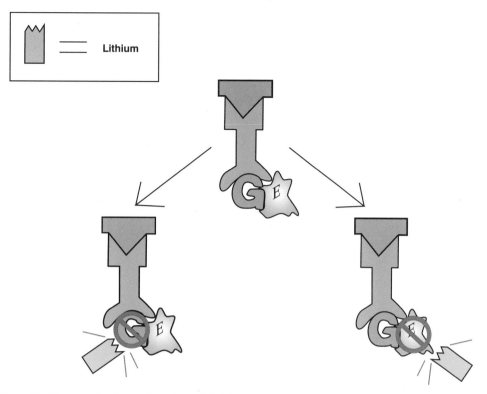

FIGURE 3–22. The **mechanism of action of lithium** is not well understood but is hypothesized to involve **modifying second messenger systems**. One possibility is that lithium alters **G proteins** and their ability to transduce signals inside the cell once the neurotransmitter receptor is occupied by the neurotransmitter. Another theory is that lithium alters **enzymes** that interact with the second-messenger system, such as inositol monophosphatase, or others.

such as dyspepsia, nausea, vomiting, and diarrhea, as well as weight gain, hair loss, acne, tremor, sedation, decreased cognition, and incoordination. There are also long-term adverse effects on the thyroid and kidney. Lithium has a narrow therapeutic window, requiring monitoring of plasma drug levels.

Anticonvulsants as Mood Stabilizers

Based on theories that mania may "kindle" further episodes of mania, a logical parallel with seizure disorders was drawn, since seizures can kindle more seizures. Thus, trials of several anticonvulsants, beginning with carbamazepine, have been conducted, and several are showing indications of efficacy in treating the manic phase of bipolar disorder (Table 3–1). Only valproic acid, however, is actually approved for this indication.

The mechanism of action of anticonvulsants remains poorly characterized, both in terms of their anticonvulsant effects or their antimanic/mood stabilizing effects. They may even have multiple mechanisms of action. At the cell membrane, anti-convulsants appear to act on ion channels, including sodium, potassium, and calcium channels. By interfering with sodium movements through voltage-operated sodium

Table 3–1. *Anticonvulsants used
to treat bipolar disorder*

valproic acid (Depakote)
carbamazepine
lamotrigine
gabapentin
topiramate

channels, for example, several anticonvulsants cause use-dependent blockade of sodium inflow. That is, when the sodium channels are being "used" during neuronal activity such as seizures, anticonvulsants can prolong their inactivation, thus providing anticonvulsant action. Whether such a mechanism is also the cause of the mood-stabilizing effects of anticonvulsants is yet unknown.

When ion channels are inactivated, this may result in changes of both excitatory and inhibitory neurotransmission. Glutamate is the universal excitatory neurotransmitter and gamma-aminobutyric acid (GABA) is the universal inhibitory neurotransmitter. In particular, anticonvulsants appear to modulate the effects of the inhibitory neurotransmitter GABA by augmenting its synthesis, augmenting its release, inhibiting its breakdown, reducing its reuptake into GABA neurons, or augmenting its effects at GABA receptors. Some of these actions may be the consequence of anticonvulsant actions at ion channels.

Anticonvulsants may also interfere with neurotransmission by the excitatory neurotransmitter glutamate, in particular by reducing its release. Simply put, inhibitory neurotransmission with GABA may be enhanced and excitatory neurotransmission with glutamate may be reduced by anticonvulsants.

Other actions of some anticonvulsants include inhibition of the enzyme carbonic anhydrase, negative modulation of calcium channel activity, and actions on second messenger systems, including inhibition of phosphokinase C. Beyond the second messenger, there is the possibility that second messenger systems may be affected, analogously to what is hypothesized for lithium.

Valproic acid. Although its exact mechanism of action remains uncertain, valproic acid (also valproate sodium, or valproate) may inhibit sodium and/or calcium channel function and perhaps thereby boost GABA inhibitory action as well as reduce glutamate excitatory action (Fig. 3–23). A unique and patented pharmaceutical formulation of valproic acid, called Depakote, reduces gastrointestinal side effects.

The Depakote form of valproic acid is approved for the acute phase of bipolar disorder. It is also commonly used on a long-term basis, although its prophylactic effects have not been as well established. Valproic acid is now frequently used as a first-line treatment for bipolar disorders, as well as in combination with lithium for patients refractory to lithium monotherapy and especially for patients with rapid cycling and mixed episodes. Oral loading can lead to rapid stabilization, and plasma levels must be monitored to keep drug levels within the therapeutic range.

Valproic acid can have unacceptable side effects, such as hair loss, weight gain, and sedation. Certain problems can limit valproic acid's usefulness in women of child-bearing potential, including the fact that it can cause neural tube defects in

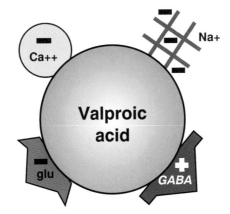

FIGURE 3–23. Shown here is an icon of **valproic acid**'s pharmacologic actions. By interfering with calcium channels and sodium channels, valproate is thought both to enhance the inhibitory actions of gamma aminobutyric acid (GABA) and to reduce the excitatory actions of glutamate.

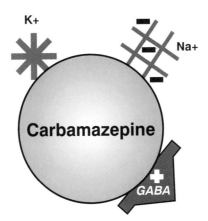

FIGURE 3–24. Shown here is an icon of **carbamazepine**'s pharmacologic actions. By interfering with sodium and potassium, carbamazepine is thought to enhance the inhibitory actions of gamma aminobutyric acid (GABA).

the developing fetus. Menstrual disturbances, polycystic ovaries, hyperandrogenism, obesity, and insulin resistance may also be associated with valproic acid therapy.

Carbamazepine. The anticonvulsant carbamazepine was actually the first to be shown to be effective in the manic phase of bipolar disorder, but it has not been approved for this use by regulatory authorities such as the U.S. Food and Drug Administration (FDA). Its mechanism of action may be to enhance GABA function, perhaps in part by actions on sodium and/or potassium channels (Fig. 3–24). Because its efficacy is less well documented and its side effects can include sedation and hematological abnormalities, it is not as well accepted for first-line use in the treatment of mood disorders as either lithium or valproic acid.

Lamotrigine. Lamotrigine is approved as an anticonvulsant but not as a mood stabilizer. It is postulated to inhibit sodium channels and to inhibit the release of glu-

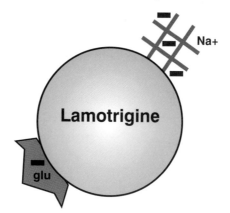

FIGURE 3–25. Shown here is an icon of **lamotrigine**'s pharmacologic actions. By interfering with sodium channels, lamotrigine is thought to reduce the excitatory actions of glutamate.

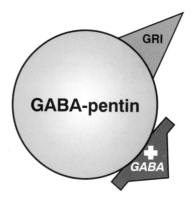

FIGURE 3–26. Shown here is an icon of **gabapentin**'s pharmacologic actions. Gabapentin is thought to act by inhibiting the reuptake of gamma aminobutyric acid (GABA) into GABA terminals (shown as GRI for GABA reuptake inhibition). This enhances the inhibitory actions of GABA.

tamate (Fig. 3–25). Numerous reports suggest that lamotrigine is not only able to stabilize bipolar manic and mixed episodes but it may also be useful for the depressive episodes of this disorder. Further testing of lamotrigine's safety and efficacy in mood disorders is ongoing.

Gabapentin. This compound was synthesized as a GABA analogue but turned out not to directly modulate the GABA receptor. It may well interact at the GABA transporter and increase GABA levels (Fig. 3–26). It also decreases glutamate levels. It is approved as an anticonvulsant and was originally observed to improve mood and quality of life in seizure disorder patients. Numerous studies suggest efficacy in the manic phase of bipolar disorder, and further clinical evaluation as a mood stabilizer is ongoing. A gabapentin analogue called pregabalin is also undergoing clinical evaluation as an anticonvulsant and as a mood stabilizer.

Topiramate. Topiramate is another compound approved as an anticonvulsant and in clinical testing as a mood stabilizer. Its mechanism of action appears to be to enhance

GABA function and reduce glutamate function by interfering with both sodium and calcium channels. In addition, it is a weak inhibitor of carbonic anhydrase (Fig. 3–27). Topiramate's mood-stabilizing actions may occur at lower doses than its anticonvulsant actions. This compound also has the interesting side effect of weight loss in some patients, a most unique effect among mood stabilizers, which generally cause weight gain.

Other Mood Stabilizing Drugs

Benzodiazepines. Benzodiazepines have anticonvulsant actions, especially intravenous diazepam and oral clonazepam. They are also sedating. Both of these actions have led to the use of benzodiazepines for the treatment of mood disorders, especially as adjunctive treatment for agitation and psychotic behavior during the phase of acute mania. Benzodiazepines are also broadly used in anxiety and sleep disorders.

Antipsychotics. Classical neuroleptics (such as helperidol and the phenothiazine chlorpromazine) have long played a role in the treatment of agitation and the psychosis of mania. More recently, the atypical antipsychotics (such as risperidone, olanzapine and guetiapine) have begun to replace the older neuroleptics and assume an important adjunctive role in the treatment of bipolar disorders. Atypical antipsychotics may also improve mood in schizophrenia. Currently, the atypical antipsychotics are becoming more widely used for management of the manic phase of bipolar disorder. Clinical studies are also ongoing to determine the role of these agents in the long-term management of bipolar disorder, including first-line use, maintenance treatment, and use in combination with mood stabilizers for treatment-resistant cases, especially mixed and rapid cycling cases.

Drug Combinations for Treatment-Resistant Patients— Rational Polypharmacy

So far, we have discussed many individual members of the "depression pharmacy" (Fig. 3–28). More than two dozen different agents acting by eight distinct mechanisms are thus useful for treating the typical case of depression (Fig. 3–29). However, psychopharmacologists are increasingly being called on to provide treatment for patients who do not respond to their initial treatment with one or another of the various antidepressants available from the depression pharmacy (Figs. 3–28 and 3–29). The following section is a somewhat complex discussion of how different drugs are combined to treat depression and bipolar disorders, and may not be of interest to the novice. Thus, some readers may wish to skip this section and jump ahead to the section on electroconvulsive therapy.

The most frequent strategy for managing patients who do not respond to several different antidepressant monotherapies is to augment treatment with a second agent. Such treatment-resistant (sometimes also called treatment-refractory) cases have classically been approached with an algorithm, first trying single agents from different pharmacological classes (Fig. 3–29) and then boosting single agents with a second drug, making for a variety of possible drug combinations (Figs. 3–30 through 3–57). The three augmenting agents that have been most studied are lithium, thyroid hormone, and buspirone. Other augmenting strategies discussed here are commonly

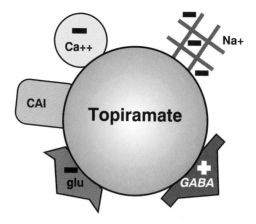

FIGURE 3–27. Shown here is an icon of **topiramate**'s pharmacologic actions. By interfering with calcium channels and sodium channels, topiramate is thought both to enhance the inhibitory actions of gamma aminobutyric acid (GABA) and to reduce the excitatory actions of glutamate. Topiramate is also a carbonic anhydrase inhibitor (CAI) and as such has independent anticonvulsant actions.

employed in practice, but their use is often based more on art and anecdote than on scientific studies.

Lithium and Mood Stabilizers as Augmenting Agents

Lithium is the classical augmenting agent for unipolar depression resistant to first-line treatment with antidepressants (classic combo in Fig. 7–30). Lithium may boost the antidepressant actions of first-line antidepressants by acting synergistically on second messenger systems. Early studies indicate that the anticonvulsant class of mood stabilizers can also augment inadequate treatment responses to first-line antidepressants. Lithium and anticonvulsants are also used in combination with antidepressants for bipolar depression; however, in this disorder the mood stabilizers are the first-line treatment and antidepressants are given to augment inadequate response to a mood stabilizer rather than the other way around (see discussion of combination treatments for bipolar disorders below).

Thyroid Hormone as an Augmenting Agent

Since thyroid illness is commonly associated with depression, especially in women, it has long been observed that treating the thyroid abnormalities also can reverse the depression. This is especially true for treating hypothyroidism with thyroid hormone replacement (either T3 or T4). It has even been observed that giving supplemental thyroid hormone to depressed patients unresponsive to first-line antidepressants but without overt hypothyroidism can boost the antidepressant response of the first-line antidepressant (thyroid combo in Fig. 3–30). Thyroid hormone is also commonly administered to bipolar patients resistant to mood stabilizers, particularly those with rapid cycling (see discussion of combinations for bipolar disorders below).

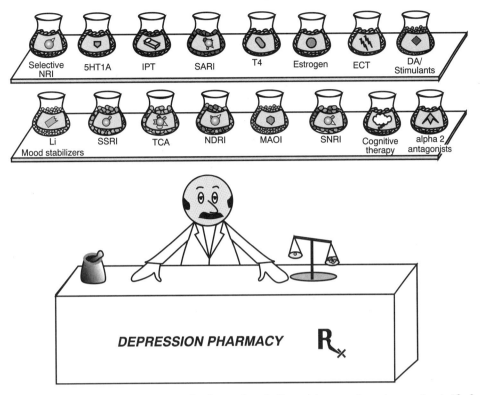

FIGURE 3–28. There are many treatments for depression, indicated here as therapies on the shelf of the depression pharmacy. Many of these treatments are used as single interventions in the treatment of depression. The therapies include **selective norepinephrine reuptake inhibitors** (selective NRIs); serotonin 1A receptor agonists (**5HT1A agents**) interpersonal psychotherapy (IPT); serotonin antagonists/reuptake inhibitors (**SARIs**); thyroid hormone (**TH**) or **estrogen**; electroconvulsive therapy (**ECT**); dopaminergic agonists such as pramipexole and dopamine releasers/stimulants such as amphetamine and methylphenidate **DA/stimulants**; lithium (**Li**) or other mood stabilizers; serotonin selective reuptake inhibitors (**SSRIs**); tricyclic antidepressants (**TCAs**); norepinephrine and dopamine reuptake inhibitors (**NDRIs**); monoamine oxidase inhibitors (**MAOIs**); serotonin norepinephrine reuptake inhibitors (**SNRIs**); **cognitive therapy** (psychotherapy) and **alpha 2 antagonists**.

Buspirone, the Serotonin 1A Augmenting Agent

The serotonin 1A partial agonist buspirone, whose primary use is in generalized anxiety disorder, is also used as a popular augmenting agent for treatment-resistant depression, particularly in North America (serotonin 1A combo in Fig. 3–30). Its potential mechanism of action as an antidepressant augmenting agent is shown in Figures 3–31 to 3–33.

If serotonin is very low or depleted from serotonergic neurons in depression, there would not be much of it released for an SSRI to block its reuptake (Fig. 3–31). Thus, there would theoretically be inadequate desensitization of somatodendritic 5HT1A autoreceptors. Unlike the SSRIs, which are all dependent for their actions on the endogenous release of serotonin, buspirone is not dependent on serotonin levels because it has direct actions on 5HT1A receptors (Fig. 3–32). Thus, buspirone may be able to "kick start" the desensitization process directly. Initially,

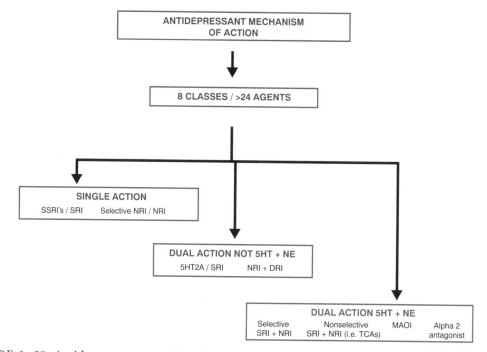

FIGURE 3–29. **Antidepressant monotherapies** organized by mechanism of action. There are over two dozen agents acting by eight distinct pharmacological mechanisms. These include antidepressants that have single neurotransmitter action (the five SSRIs and the selective NRI reboxetine); agents that have dual actions on the same or similar neurotransmitter system (the SARI nefazodone and the NDRI bupropion); and agents that have dual actions (TCAs, MAOIs, the dual SNRI venlafaxine, and the alpha 2 antagonist mirtazapine).

buspirone also slows neuronal impulses, which may also help the neuron to replete its serotonin (Fig. 3–32).

Thus, buspirone is synergistic with the SSRIs (Fig. 3–33). To the extent that buspirone is a partial agonist and thus partially blocks the 5HT1A autoreceptors, it

FIGURE 3–30. Combination treatments for unipolar depression (unipolar combos). The treatment of depression generally begins with a single agent, called a **first-line agent**, as **monotherapy**. If single agents acting by a single neurotransmitter mechanism fail, then single agents acting by multiple neurotransmitter mechanisms may be effective. If these monotherapies also fail, antidepressants are often used in **combination** with other drugs, hormones, or even other antidepressants. For example, the classical combination of agents is a first-line agent with lithium or a mood stabilizer as augmentation (**classic combo**). Another strategy is to augment a first-line agent with thyroid hormone (**thyroid combo**). Yet another approach that has been well documented to work in some cases is addition of the 5HT1A partial agonist buspirone or possibly the 5HT1A antagonist pindolol to a first-line antidepressant, especially an SSRI (**serotonin 1A combo**). A powerful if potentially dangerous combination is to use a tricyclic antidepressant and a monoamine oxidase inhibitor simultaneously (**cautious combo**). Early studies suggest that addition of reproductive hormones, especially estradiol, for women with treatment-resistant depression may be helpful in some cases (**estrogen combo**). Short-term use of sedative-hypnotics or anxiolytics may be necessary if insomnia or anxiety is persistent and cannot be managed by other strategies (**insomnia/anxiety combo**).

Unipolar Combos

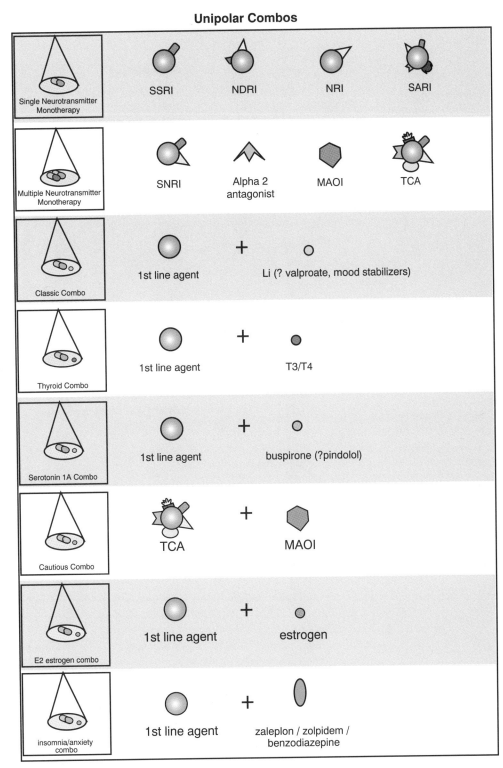

Single Neurotransmitter Monotherapy	SSRI	NDRI	NRI	SARI
Multiple Neurotransmitter Monotherapy	SNRI	Alpha 2 antagonist	MAOI	TCA
Classic Combo	1st line agent	+	Li (? valproate, mood stabilizers)	
Thyroid Combo	1st line agent	+	T3/T4	
Serotonin 1A Combo	1st line agent	+	buspirone (?pindolol)	
Cautious Combo	TCA	+	MAOI	
E2 estrogen combo	1st line agent	+	estrogen	
insomnia/anxiety combo	1st line agent	+	zaleplon / zolpidem / benzodiazepine	

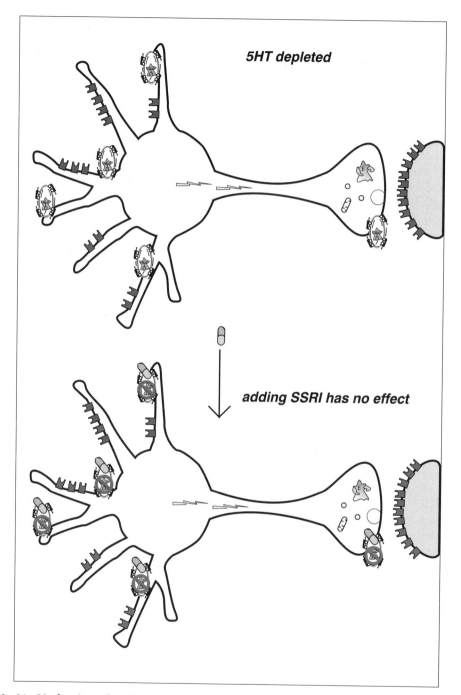

FIGURE 3–31. *Mechanism of action of buspirone augmentation*–part 1. SSRIs act indirectly by increasing synaptic levels of 5HT that has been released there. If 5HT is depleted, there is no 5HT release, and SSRIs are ineffective. This has been postulated to be the explanation for the lack of SSRI therapeutic actions or loss of therapeutic action of SSRI ("poop out") in some patients.

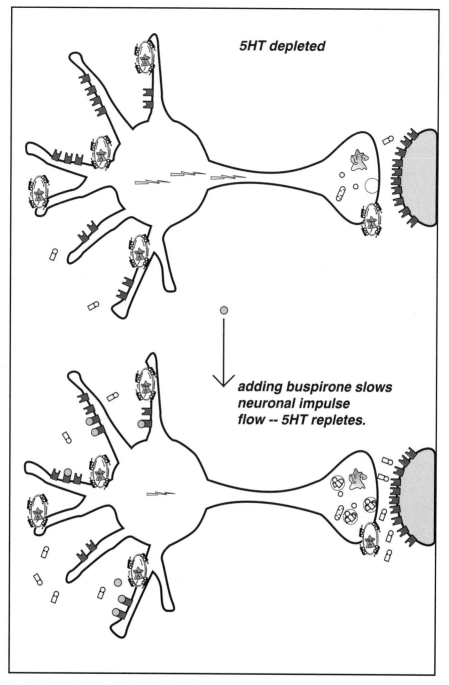

FIGURE 3–32. *Mechanism of action of buspirone augmentation–part 2.* Shown here is how buspirone may augment SSRI action both by repleting 5HT and by directly desensitizing 5HT1A receptors. One theoretical mechanism of how 5HT is allowed to reaccumulate in the 5HT-depleted neuron is the shutdown of neuronal impulse flow. If 5HT release is essentially turned off for a while so that the neuron retains all the 5HT it synthesizes, this may allow repletion of 5HT stores. A 5HT1A partial agonist such as buspirone acts directly on somatodendritic autoreceptors to inhibit neuronal impulse flow, possibly allowing repletion of 5HT stores. Also, buspirone could boost actions directly at 5HT1A receptors to help the small amount of 5HT available in this scenario accomplish the targeted desensitization of 5HT1A somatodendritic autoreceptors that is necessary for antidepressant actions.

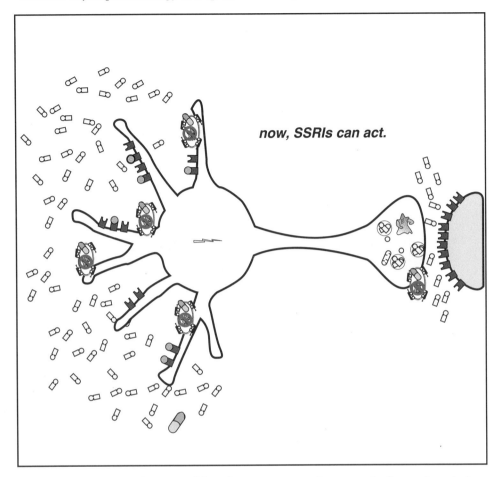

now, SSRIs can act.

FIGURE 3–33. *Mechanism of action of buspirone augmentation*–part 3. Shown here is how buspirone potentiates ineffective SSRI action at 5HT1A somatodendritic autoreceptors, resulting in the desired disinhibition of the 5HT neuron. This combination of 5HT1A agonists plus SSRIs may be more effective, not only in depression but also in other disorders treated by SSRIs, such as obsessive-compulsive disorder and panic.

may act even faster than an SSRI. Blockade of these receptors immediately disinhibits them, whereas stimulation of them causes delayed disinhibition due to the time it takes for them to desensitize.

Pindolol, Another Serotonin 1A Augmenting Agent

The idea of blocking 5HT1A somatodendritic autoreceptors is also exploited by pindolol, a well-known beta adrenergic blocker that also is an antagonist and very partial agonist at 5HT1A receptors. Preclinical studies suggest that pindolol can immediately disinhibit serotonin neurons, leading to the proposal that it may be a rapid onset antidepressant or augmenting agent. Some clinical studies do suggest that pindolol augmentation may speed the onset of action of SSRIs or may boost inadequate response to SSRIs, but not all investigators agree. Nevertheless, 5HT1A antagonists are in development as potential novel and rapid-acting antidepressants.

Monoamine Oxidase Inhibitor/Tricyclic Antidepressant Combinations

One old-fashioned augmentation strategy that has fallen out of favor in recent years is to combine with great caution a TCA and an MAO inhibitor (the cautious combo in Fig. 3–30). Given its potential dangers (e.g., sudden hypertensive episodes, orthostatic hypotension, drug and dietary interactions, obesity), as well as the wide variety of other antidepressant combinations available today, this combination is rarely necessary or justified.

Estrogen and Reproductive Hormones as Antidepressant Augmenting Agents

Another hormone combination therapy is to combine a first-line antidepressant, especially an SSRI, with estrogen replacement therapy in perimenopausal or postmenopausal women refractory to treatment with antidepressant monotherapies (the estrogen combo in Fig. 3–30). Unfortunately, there are few if any controlled clinical trials to provide guidance on how to combine estrogen with antidepressants. Numerous case reports and anecdotes from clinicians demonstrate that some women respond to estrogen who do not respond to antidepressants, and other women respond to estrogen plus an antidepressant who do not respond to antidepressants alone. Since estrogen is itself a direct activator of transcription, it may be able to synergize at the genomic level with the transcription activated by SSRIs (Fig. 3–34) to produce a molecular result greater than that which the SSRIs can produce alone.

Other uses of the reproductive hormone approach are to avoid cyclical use of estrogen/progestins, eliminate progestins, add testosterone, or add dihydroepiandrosterone (DHEA). Such approaches remain anecdotal and require controlled studies of how they may be useful augmenting agents for antidepressants both in women and in men.

Insomnia/Anxiety Combinations

Insomnia is a common comorbid condition with depression, and frequently is made worse by antidepressants, particularly the SSRIs. When insomnia persists despite adequate evaluation and attempts to reduce it by other approaches, it is often necessary to use a concomitant sedative-hypnotic, especially a short-acting nonbenzodiazepine with rapid onset such as zaleplon or zolpidem. At times a benzodiazepine sedative hypnotic such as triazolam or temazepam may be necessary. If anxiety persists during the day and cannot be otherwise managed, it may be necessary to add an anxiolytic benzodiazepine such as alprazolam or clonazepam. Use of sedative-hypnotics and anxiolytics should be short-term whenever possible.

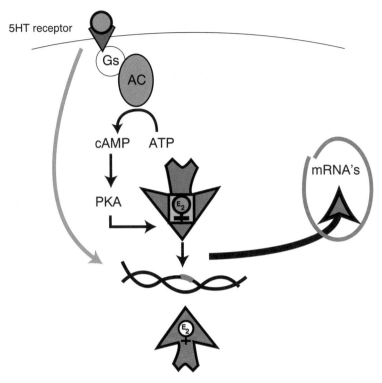

5HT receptor

Gs

AC

cAMP   ATP

PKA

mRNA's

FIGURE 3–34. **Estrogen** acts at receptors in the neuronal cell nucleus to directly **boost the transcription of genes**. This may be synergistic with the antidepressant actions of first-line antidepressant agents in activating transcription factors (TF) in some women.

Bipolar Combinations

Combination treatment with two or more psychotropic medications is the rule rather than the exception for bipolar disorders (bipolar combos in Fig. 3–35). First-line treatment is with either lithium or valproic acid. When patients fail to stabilize in the acute manic phase on one of these first-line treatments, the preferred second-

FIGURE 3–35. Combination treatments for bipolar disorder (**bipolar combos**). Combination drug treatment is the rule rather than the exception for patients with bipolar disorder. It is best to attempt monotherapy, however, with first-line lithium or valproic acid, with second-line atypical antipsychotics, or with third-line anticonvulsant mood stabilizers. A very common situation in acute treatment of the manic phase of bipolar disorder is to treat with both a mood stabilizer and an atypical antipsychotic (**atypical combo**). Agitated patients may require intermittent doses of sedating benzodiazepines (**benzo assault weapon**), whereas patients out of control may require intermittent doses of tranquilizing neuroleptics (**neuroleptic nuclear weapon**). For maintenance treatment, patients often require combinations of two mood stabilizers (**mood stabilizer combo**) or a mood stabilizer with an atypical antipsychotic (**atypical combo**). For patients who have depressive episodes despite mood stabilizer or atypical combos, antidepressants may be required (**antidepressant combo**). However, antidepressants may also decompensate patients into overt mania, rapid cycling states, or mixed states of mania and depression. Thus, antidepressant combos are used cautiously.

Bipolar Combos

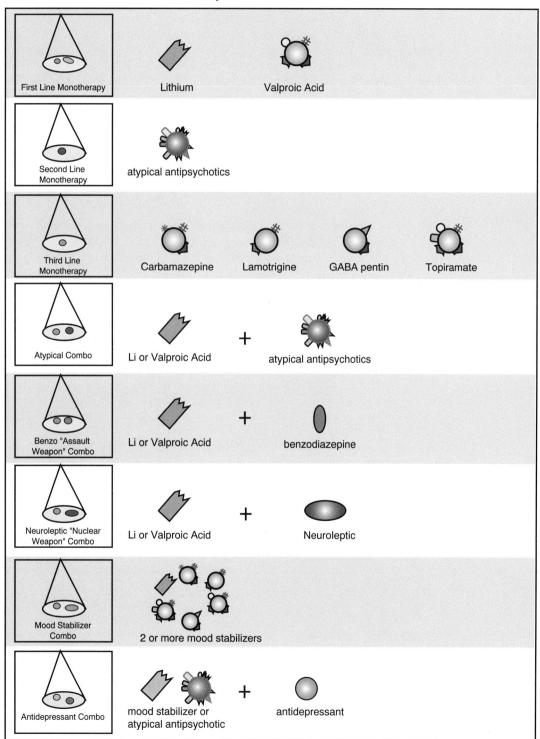

First Line Monotherapy	Lithium	Valproic Acid
Second Line Monotherapy	atypical antipsychotics	
Third Line Monotherapy	Carbamazepine Lamotrigine GABA pentin Topiramate	
Atypical Combo	Li or Valproic Acid + atypical antipsychotics	
Benzo "Assault Weapon" Combo	Li or Valproic Acid + benzodiazepine	
Neuroleptic "Nuclear Weapon" Combo	Li or Valproic Acid + Neuroleptic	
Mood Stabilizer Combo	2 or more mood stabilizers	
Antidepressant Combo	mood stabilizer or atypical antipsychotic + antidepressant	

line agent is an atypical antipsychotic. Atypical antipsychotics are even becoming first-line treatments for the manic phase of bipolar disorder.

If lithium, valproic acid, or atypical antipsychotic monotherapies are not effective in the acute situation, they can be used together (atypical combo in Fig. 3–35). If this is not effective, a benzodiazepine or a conventional antipsychotic (i.e., a neuroleptic) can be added to first- or second-line monotherapies, especially for the most disturbed patients (Fig. 3–35). That is, sedating benzodiazepines can be used for lesser degrees of agitation (benzo assault weapon in Fig. 3–35), but neuroleptic antipsychotics may be necessary for the most disturbed and out-of-control patients (nuclear weapon in Fig. 3–35). Neuroleptic antipsychotics should be restricted to the acute phase, and administered sparingly.

For maintenance treatment, failure of first-line mood stabilizers or second-line atypical antipsychotics to control symptoms adequately may lead to monotherapy trials with other anticonvulsants such as carbamazepine, lamotrigine, gabapentin, and topiramate (third-line monotherapy).

Therapeutic recommendations for maintenance treatment of bipolar disorder are undergoing rapid changes. In the recent past, lithium was the hallmark of this treatment, often with antidepressant co-therapy for patients prone to depression as well as mania and not adequately controlled by lithium alone. Now, however, several new therapeutic principles are guiding the treatment of bipolar disorders in the maintenance phase.

First, anticonvulsants, particularly valproic acid, are now considered excellent first-line choices along with lithium, although lithium is the only agent approved for such use.

Second, atypical antipsychotics are clearly second-line choices for maintenance therapy of bipolar disorder when one or more mood stabilizers alone or in combination are not adequate. Furthermore, atypical antipsychotics are also becoming first-line choices for bipolar maintenance as the safety and efficacy data from controlled trials continue to evolve.

Third, antidepressant treatments are not benign in this condition. Although many bipolar patients have been classically maintained on both lithium and an antidepressant, it is now recognized that antidepressants frequently decompensate bipolar patients, causing not only overt mania or hypomania, but also the problems of mixed mania and rapid cycling, which are much more difficult to recognize and treat. The trend today is to use antidepressants sparingly and if necessary, only in the presence of robust mood stabilization with mood stabilizers, atypical antipsychotics, or both. In fact, both mood stabilizers and atypical antipsychotics may prove to be useful for the depressed phase of bipolar illness, reducing or perhaps eliminating the need for potentially destabilizing antidepressants in bipolar patients. Thus, antidepressants are now relegated to third-line use in bipolar disorder, behind lithium or anticonvulsant mood stabilizers and atypical antipsychotics. This is an antidepressant-sparing strategy for the treatment of bipolar disorder.

Combination treatments for maintenance of bipolar disorder can include two or more mood stabilizers; a mood stabilizer and an atypical antipsychotic; a mood stabilizer and/or atypical antipsychotic with a benzodiazepine; a mood stabilizer with thyroid hormone; and even a mood stabilizer and/or atypical antipsychotic with an antidepressant (Fig. 3–35).

A Rational Approach to Antidepressant Combinations with Other Antidepressants

In the current managed care era, the modern psychopharmacologist/psychiatrist may deal almost exclusively with patients resistant to conventional treatment approaches, since easier cases are handled by lower cost or primary care providers, and these difficult cases are selectively referred. Treating patients resistant to well documented strategies by using less well documented but pharmacologically and molecularly rational strategies is not for the novice, nor for those who wish to work within treatment guidelines for drugs with government regulatory approvals and with the documentation of numerous published controlled clinical trials. First-line mono-therapies and combination therapies are summarized in Figure 3–36.

The rationale for proceeding to the use of combinations of two antidepressants is based on a number of factors. First, certain combinations of antidepressants can exploit theoretical pharmacologic and molecular synergies to boost monoaminergic neurotransmission. Second, some combinations of antidepressants have anecdotal and empirical evidence of safety and efficacy from uncontrolled use in clinical practice. Finally, the idea of using multiple pharmacologic mechanisms simultaneously for the most difficult cases is already a recognized therapeutic approach in other areas of medicine, such as the treatment of resistant bacterial and human immunodeficiency virus infections, cancer, and resistant hypertension. Later in this chapter we will describe three specific approaches to the management of patients resistant to first-line monotherapies and typical augmentation strategies, namely, the seroto-nergic strategy, the adrenergic strategy, and the dual-mechanism or "heroic" strategy.

Diagnosing treatment resistance. Many patients have a difficult time with antidepressants, and following a trial with several of drugs, it is easy to conclude that they are treatment-resistant. Prior to concluding that a patient is not responding to antidepressants and therefore truly treatment-resistant, however, it is necessary to carefully review the treatment history to rule out medication intolerance masquerading as medication resistance (e.g., many medications tried, but few adequate trials of full doses for 4 to 8 weeks). The solution to medication intolerance may be to augment with an antidepressant that cancels the side effects of the antidepressant that is not tolerable.

The other situation to rule out when establishing treatment resistance in depression is misdiagnosis as resistant unipolar depression when the patient is actually bipolar. That is, an apparently unipolar patient with drug-induced agitation may actually be a bipolar patient with antidepressant-induced rapid cycling or mixed mania of an unrecognized bipolar disorder. This situation will commonly be exacerbated by combining two antidepressants. The solution to this problem may, in fact, be to discontinue antidepressants and optimize treatment with mood stabilizers and atypical antipsychotics before using any antidepressant agent.

Principles of antidepressant combinations. The first principle of combination treatment with antidepressants is to combine mechanisms, not just drugs. That is, the important thing is the pharmacological mechanisms being combined; drugs are just the "mules" that carry mechanisms on their backs. Some drugs have one principal mech-

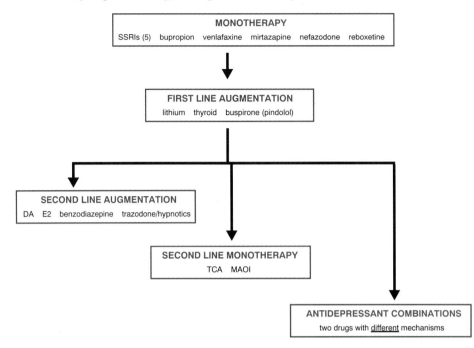

FIGURE 3–36. This figure summarizes both **first-line monotherapies** and the most commonly used **combination therapies** for unipolar depression. Note that antidepressant combinations at the far right and the end of the line are to be used after other strategies fail.

anism, others multiple mechanisms. Thus, combining two drugs may in fact be combining three or more mechanisms. Furthermore, there are many different drug mules that carry the same mechanisms, allowing for multiple approaches to achieving any given mixture of mechanisms by using several different combinations of drugs.

A second principle of antidepressant combination is to promote bad mathematics. That is, successful mixture of drug mechanisms leads to pharmacological synergy for antidepressant therapeutic actions (where 1 + 1 = 10). Furthermore, knowing the mechanism of antidepressant side effects can lead to other successful mixtures of drug mechanisms where opposing side effect profiles promote tolerability (in other words, where 1 + 1 = 0). The cleverest mixtures of antidepressants can yield both forms of bad mathematics at the same time, namely synergistic boost to efficacy along with improved tolerability achieved by canceling mutual side effects.

The third principle of antidepressant combinations is to exploit theoretically important synergies within the serotonin, norepinephrine, and even dopamine monoaminergic systems. Specifically, two independent pharmacologic actions at any one of the monoaminergic systems can be synergistic. Examples of this are combination of either serotonin or norepinephrine reuptake blockade with alpha 2 blockade, or 5HT reuptake blockade with serotonin 2A antagonism, as discussed earlier in this chapter. Specific examples of how to implement this approach for serotonin are given in Figure 3–37. Specific examples of how to implement this approach for norepinephrine and dopamine are given in Figures 3–38 to 3–43.

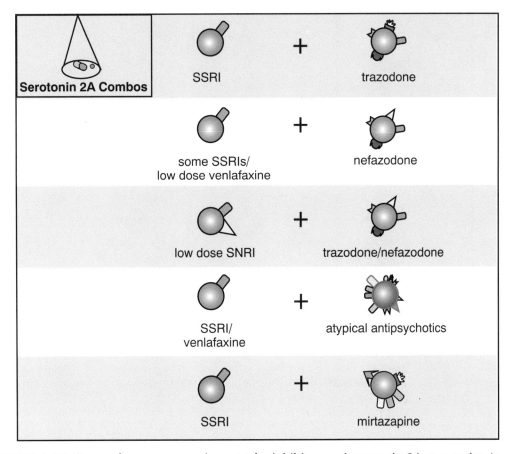

Serotonin 2A Combos	SSRI	+	trazodone
	some SSRIs/ low dose venlafaxine	+	nefazodone
	low dose SNRI	+	trazodone/nefazodone
	SSRI/ venlafaxine	+	atypical antipsychotics
	SSRI	+	mirtazapine

FIGURE 3–37. Synergy between **serotonin reuptake inhibitors** and **serotonin 2A antagonists** is commonly observed. Various specific drug combinations to implement this strategy in unipolar depression are shown here.

The other theoretically important synergy to exploit for treating resistant depression is that between serotonin and norepinephrine (e.g., Figs. 3–39 and 3–44). Thus, boosting neurotransmission at both monoamine systems with either a single drug or combinations of drugs can also boost therapeutic efficacy in treatment-resistant depression. Several specific examples of how to implement this strategy are given in Figures 3–45 to 3–57.

Synergy within the serotoninergic system. Boosting serotonin neurotransmission has proved to be useful not only in treatment-resistant depression, but for treatment resistance within the whole family of "serotonin spectrum disorders," such as obsessive-compulsive disorder, panic disorder, social phobia, posttraumatic stress disorder, and bulimia.

A major example of pharmacologic synergy within the serotonin system is the 5HT2A antagonist strategy. This is shown in Figures 3–20 and 3–21 and was discussed earlier in the section on nefazodone and the SARIs. For this strategy, robust inhibition of serotonin reuptake by agents in the left column of Figure 3–37 is

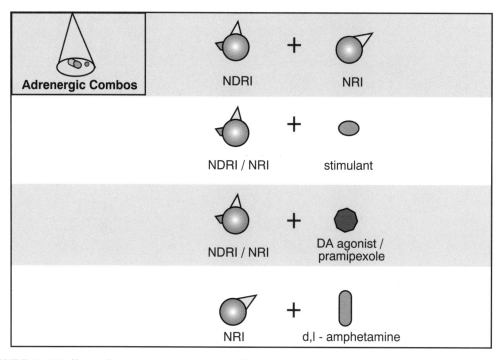

FIGURE 3–38. Shown here are various drug combinations for use in treatment resistant unipolar depression to **boost adrenergic neurotransmission**, which include either norepinephrine, dopamine, or both.

combined with robust inhibition of serotonin 2A receptors in the right column of Figure 3–37. These are not necessarily the only mechanisms combined by the specific agents shown, but this strategy is the common denominator across all pairings.

Perhaps the most commonly used example of the serotonin 2A strategy is the combination of an SSRI with trazodone. Clinicians have long recognized that trazodone will improve the agitation and insomnia often associated with SSRIs, allow high doses of the SSRI to be given, and consequently boost the efficacy of the SSRI not only in depression, but also in obsessive-compulsive disorder and other anxiety disorders. Thus, both types of bad math are in play here.

Perhaps the best documented example showing the enhanced efficacy of this serotonin 2A antagonist strategy is the use of the atypical antipsychotics to boost efficacy in nonpsychotic depression refractory to treatment with an SSRI.

Norepinephrine and synergy. Boosting noradrenergic neurotransmission may be useful not only in depression in general, but in partial responders as well, especially those with fatigue, apathy, and cognitive slowing. Several examples of how to boost noradrenergic neurotransmission beyond that of single agents alone are given in Figure 3–38. Thus, selective noradrenergic reuptake inhibitors such as reboxetine or nonselective noradrenergic reuptake inhibitors such as desipramine can be combined with the noradrenergic/dopaminergic agent bupropion. Also, bupropion or a noradrenergic reuptake inhibitor can be combined with a dopamine-releasing stimulant (such as amphetamine, methylphenidate, diethylpropion or phentermine) or with a

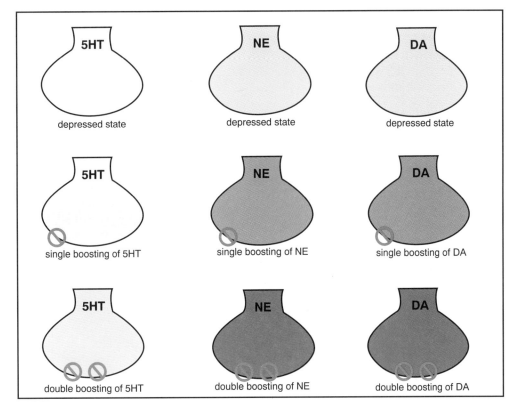

FIGURE 3–39. **Key to combos.** The figures from here to the end of the chapter will employ the visual key shown here. The depressed, unmedicated state is shown by faded colors representing neurotransmitter depletion. If any of the three monoamine neurotransmitters (5HT, NE, or DA) is boosted by one of the drugs in the combination being illustrated, its corresponding color will light up moderately. Thus, single boosting of 5HT will moderately light up yellow; single boosting of NE will moderately light up purple; and single boosting of DA will moderately light up blue. Some of the combos have synergistic actions on the same monoamine neurotransmitter system. In such cases, the colors will be doubly lit up to represent the potential synergy of this approach by the brightest coloring of 5HT (yellow), NE (purple), or DA (blue).

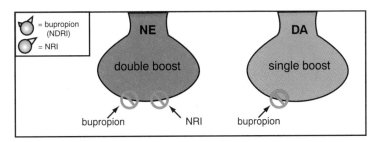

FIGURE 3–40. **Adrenergic combo 1: Bupropion** plus norepinephrine reuptake inhibitor (**NRI**). Here the NE actions of bupropion are double-boosted by the NRI (either selective reboxetine or nonselective desipramine, maprotilene, nortriptyline, or protriptyline). Dopamine is single-boosted by bupropion only.

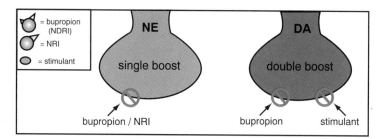

FIGURE 3–41. **Adrenergic combo 2: Bupropion** can be combined with a **stimulant** such as *d*-amphetamine or methylphenidate. The stimulant will add a double dopamine boost to bupropion, which boosts dopamine in its own right. A single boost of norepinephrine from bupropion also is present.

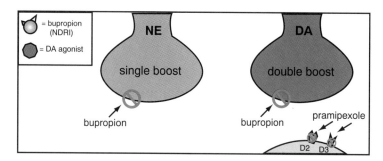

FIGURE 3–42. **Adrenergic combo 3:** The actions of **bupropion** at dopamine neurons can be double-boosted by a direct-acting dopamine **D2 and D3 agonist** such as pramipexole. Norepinephrine is also single-boosted by bupropion.

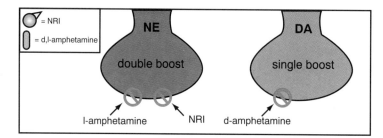

FIGURE 3–43. **Adrenergic combo 4: NRI** plus *d,l*-amphetamine. In this case, the NRI action at NE is double-boosted by a mixture of amphetamine salts containing the *l* as well as the *d* form of amphetamine. The *l*-amphetamine causes NE release. In addition, DA will be single-boosted by the *d*-amphetamine, which causes DA release.

direct dopamine agonist such as pramipexole. Anecdotally, this may be especially useful for patients with retarded or melancholic depression or those who require an antidepressant concomitantly with a mood stabilizer for bipolar depression.

The heroic strategy: boosting both serotonin and norepinephrine. In the most refractory of all patients, it may be necessary to use both serotonin and adrenergic combination

Unipolar Combos

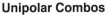

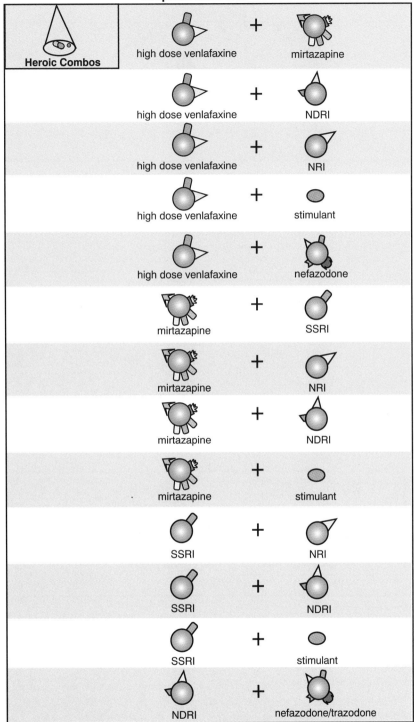

FIGURE 3–44. A baker's dozen of **heroic combos** of two antidepressants for treatment-resistant unipolar depression are shown here. Each individual-combination is explained in the figures that follow (Figs. 3–45 through 3–57).

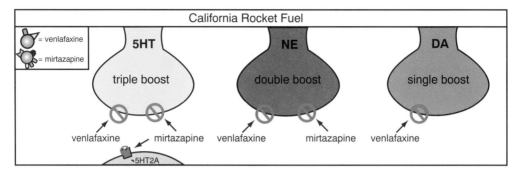

FIGURE 3–45. Heroic combo 1, or **"California rocket fuel": High-dose venlafaxine plus mirta-zapine.** This is a combination of antidepressants that has a great degree of theoretical synergy: reuptake blockade plus alpha 2 blockade; serotonin reuptake plus 5HT2A antagonism; 5HT actions plus NE actions. Specifically, 5HT is triple-boosted, with reuptake blockade, alpha 2 antagonism, and 5HT2A antagonism; NE is double-boosted, with reuptake blockade plus alpha 2 antagonism; and there may even be a bit of single boost to DA from reuptake blockade.

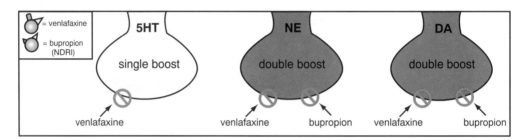

FIGURE 3–46. Heroic combo 2: **High-dose venlafaxine plus NDRI** (bupropion). Here, 5HT is single-boosted, NE is double-boosted, and DA is double-boosted.

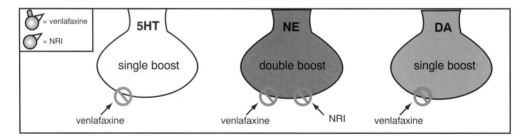

FIGURE 3–47. Heroic combo 3: **High-dose venlafaxine plus NRI.** Here, 5HT is single-boosted, NE is double-boosted, and DA may be single-boosted. The NRI could be either selective reboxetine or a nonselective TCA such as desipramine, maprotilene, nortriptyline, or protriptyline.

strategies (heroic combo; Fig. 3–44). A baker's dozen of heroic combos are given in Figure 3–44 and shown graphically in Figures 3–45 through 3–57. These specific drug combinations all do the same thing to one extent or another, namely, boost or double-boost serotonin, norepinephrine, and/or dopamine. The net effects of these combinations are shown in different shades of color in Figures 3–45 through 3–57, with light colors representing no boost to the corresponding monoamine's neuro-

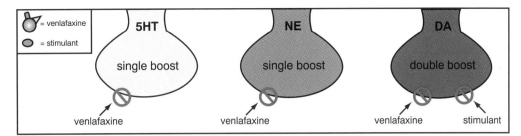

FIGURE 3–48. Heroic combo 4: **High-dose venlafaxine plus stimulant**. Here, 5HT and NE are single-boosted and DA is double-boosted. The stimulants could include *d*-amphetamine, methylphenidate, phentermine, or diethylpropion. It could also include direct-acting dopamine agonists such as pramipexole.

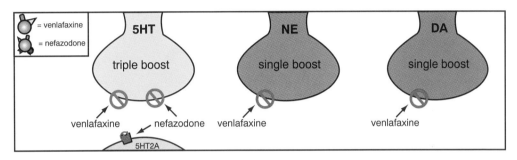

FIGURE 3–49. Heroic combo 5: **Venlafaxine plus nefazodone**. Serotonin will be double-boosted to a certain extent by nefazodone alone. At any dose of venlafaxine, the boosting of serotonin will be considerably enhanced. This enhancement of nefazodone's serotonin action can also be replicated by SSRIs, but citalopram may be the best tolerated. At high doses of venlafaxine, there will be not only boosting of 5HT but also single-boosting of NE and maybe DA.

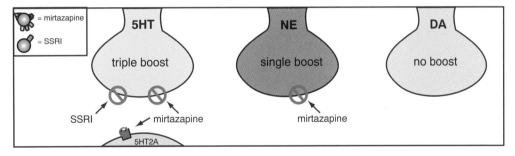

FIGURE 3–50. Heroic combo 6: **Mirtazapine plus SSRI**. Here serotonin is double-disinhibited both by reuptake blockage and by alpha 2 antagonism; NE is also single-boosted.

transmission, medium-intensity colors representing a single boost to that monoamine's neurotransmission, and high-intensity colors representing a double boost (see figure key in Fig. 3–39). One of the most theoretically powerful combinations is that of high-dose venlafaxine with mirtazapine ("California rocket fuel" in Fig. 3–45; also Fig. 3–44). These drugs combine synergies on synergy, that is, reuptake

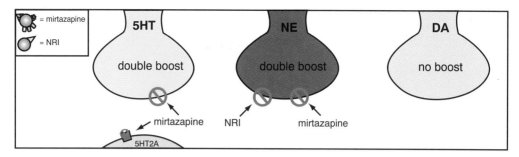

FIGURE 3–51. Heroic combo 7: **Mirtazapine plus NRI.** Here NE is double-disinhibited both by reuptake blockade and by alpha 2 antagonism. Reboxetine is better tolerated with mirtazapine than TCAs for this purpose. Serotonin is also single-boosted.

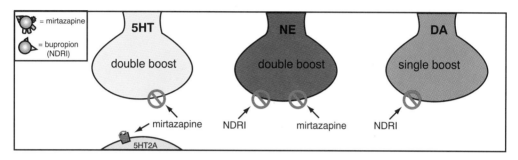

FIGURE 3–52. Heroic combo 8: **Mirtazapine plus NDRI** (bupropion). Here NE is double-boosted, and 5HT and DA are single-boosted.

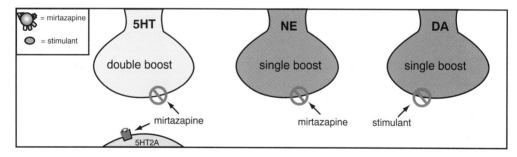

FIGURE 3–53. Heroic combo 9: **Mirtazapine plus stimulant.** Here, 5HT, NE, and DA are all single-boosted. The stimulants could include *d*-amphetamine, methylphenidate, phentermine, or di-ethylpropion. It could also include direct-acting dopamine agonists such as pramipexole.

blockade plus alpha 2 blockade for double disinhibition, actions at 5HT and NE actions boosting 5HT at 5HT1A receptors yet blocking 5HT2A receptors.

The point is to use safe and rational drug combinations that exploit expected pharmacological and molecular synergies while even promoting mutual tolerabilities. Each of the combinations in Figure 3–44 is used clinically and has helped some patients but not others. Unfortunately, little scientific documentation of this empirical usefulness of such rational combinations is yet available, but many studies

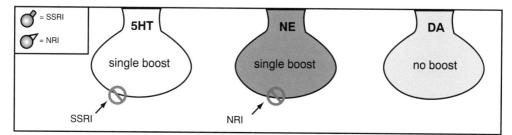

FIGURE 3–54. Heroic combo 10: **SSRI plus NRI.** Here, 5HT and NE are both single-boosted. The preferred NRI is selective reboxetine, as there are no drug interactions. Nonselective TCAs that are preferential NRIs such as desipramine, maprotilene, nortriptyline, or protriptyline can be combined if plasma drug levels of the TCA are monitored, especially if fluoxetine or paroxetine is the SSRI chosen.

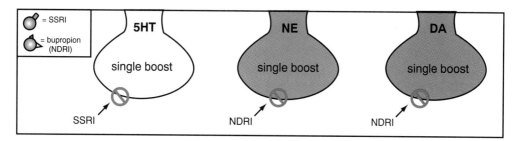

FIGURE 3–55. Heroic combo 11: **SSRI plus NDRI** (bupropion). Here 5HT, NE, and DA are all single-boosted.

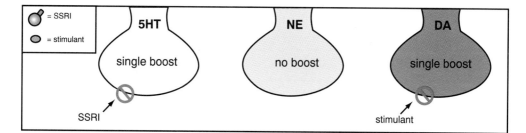

FIGURE 3–56. Heroic combo 12: **SSRI plus stimulant.** Here, 5HT and DA are single-boosted. The stimulants could include *d*-amphetamine, methylphenidate, phentermine, or diethylpropion. The combo could also include direct-acting dopamine agonists such as pramipexole.

are ongoing and should clarify the best options for the most difficult cases in which the benefits of this approach outweigh the risks.

Electroconvulsive Therapy

Failure to respond to a variety of antidepressants, singly or in combination, is the key factor indicating consideration of electroconvulsive therapy (ECT). This is the only therapeutic agent for the treatment of depression that is rapid in onset and can

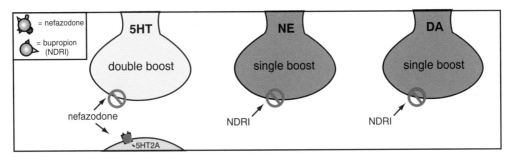

FIGURE 3–57. Heroic combo 13: **Nefazodone plus NDRI** (bupropion). In this case, the serotonergic single boost of nefazodone is added to the NE and DA single boost of bupropion.

start after even a single treatment, typically within a few days. The mechanism is unknown but is thought to be related to the probable mobilization of neurotransmitters caused by the seizure. In experimental animals, ECT down-regulates beta receptors (analogous to antidepressants) but up-regulates 5HT2 receptors (opposite of antidepressants). Memory loss and social stigma are the primary problems associated with ECT and limit its use. There can also be striking regional differences across the various countries in the world in the frequency of ECT use and in ECT techniques. For example, ECT may be more commonly used in Europe and the United Kingdom and on the U.S. East Coast and less commonly used on the U.S. West Coast.

Electroconvulsive therapy is especially useful when rapid onset of clinical effect is desired and when patients are refractory to a number of antidepressant drugs. It is also very helpful in psychotic and bipolar depression and in postpartum psychosis. If the mechanism of the therapeutic action of ECT could be unraveled, it might lead to a new antidepressant drug capable of rapid onset of antidepressant effects or with special value for refractory patients. Until then, ECT will remain a valuable member of the therapeutic armamentarium for depression.

Psychotherapy

In recent years, modern psychotherapy research has begun to standardize and test selected psychotherapies in a manner analogous to the testing of antidepresssant drugs in clinical trials. Thus, psychotherapies are now being tested by being administered according to standard protocols by therapists receiving standardized training and using standardized manuals, and also in standard "doses" for fixed duration. Such uses of psychotherapies are being compared in clinical trials with placebo or antidepressants. The results have shown that interpersonal psychotherapy and cognitive psychotherapy for depression may be as effective as antidepressants themselves in certain patients. Proof of the efficacy of certain psychotherapies is thus beginning to evolve.

Research is only beginning on how to combine psychotherapy with drugs. Although some of the earliest studies did not indicate any additive benefit of tricyclic antidepressants and interpersonal psychotherapy, recent studies are now demonstrating that there can be an additive benefit between psychotherapy and antidepressants. One recent study of nefazodone suggests that it is particularly effective when combined with cognitive behavioral psychotherapy for patients with chronic depression. Another study of nortriptyline suggests an additive benefit of interpersonal psychotherapy, particularly when looking at long-term outcomes. It is not known whether the addition of psychotherapy to antidepressant responders who are not in full remission might lead to remission and recovery, but this is an interesting possibility. Although psychotherapy is frequently employed on an empirical basis, it is not yet proven that its addition to the psychopharmacological treatment of patients resistant to antidepressant monotherapy treatment (either no response, or a response but not a remission) improves outcomes. As managed care reduces the availability of psychotherapy, mental health professionals are becoming increasingly dependent on a psychopharmacological approach. The rapidly evolving scientific demonstration of the benefit of adjunctive psychotherapy should provide much needed and welcome justification by showing who benefits from what kinds of psychotherapy combined with which specific antidepressants. Cognitive and behavioral psychotherapies are also of value as adjuncts to antidepressants for the treatment of anxiety disorders.

Summary

In this chapter, we have discussed the mechanisms of action of several of the newer classes of antidepressant drugs and mood stabilizers. The acute pharmacological actions of these agents on neurotransmitter receptors have been described. The reader should now understand the proposed mechanisms of action of dual reuptake inhibitors, alpha 2 antagonists, and serotonin 2A antagonists/serotonin reuptake inhibitors, as well as those of lithium and the anticonvulsant mood stabilizers for the treatment of bipolar disorder, particularly the acute manic phase.

We have reviewed antidepressant augmentation strategies, including the principles and several specific examples. Finally, we have touched on the use of electroconvulsive therapy and psychotherapy for the treatment of depression.

Although the specific pragmatic guidelines for use of these various therapeutic modalities for depression have not been emphasized, the reader should now have a basis for the rational use of antidepressant and mood-stabilizing drugs founded on application of principles of drug action on neurotransmission via actions at key receptors and enzymes.

SUGGESTED READING

Bloom, F.E., and Kupfer, D.J. (Eds.) (1995) *Psychopharmacology: the fourth generation of progress.* New York, Raven Press.

Bond, A.J., and Lader, M.H. (1996) *Understanding drug treatment in mental health care.* Chichester, John Wiley & Sons.

Carey, P.J., Alexander, B., and Liskow, B.I. (1997) *Psychotropic drug handbook.* Washington, DC, American Psychiatric Press.

Cooper, J.R., Bloom, F.E., and Roth, R.H. (1996) *The biochemical basis of neuropharmacology*, 7th edition. New York, Oxford University Press.

Depression in primary care, volume 1, detection and diagnosis; clinical practice guideline, number 5, U.S. Department of Health and Human Services, AHCPR Publication No. 93-0551, Public Health Service, Agency for Health Care Policy and Research, Rockville, MD, April, 1993.

Depression in primary care, volume 2, treatment of major depression; clinical practice guideline, number 5, U.S. Department of Health and Human Services, AHCPR Publication No. 93-0551, Public Health Service, Agency for Health Care Policy and Research, Rockville, MD, April, 1993.

Diagnostic and statistical manual of mental disorders, 4th edition (DSM-IV), American Psychiatric Association Press, Washington, DC, 1994.

Dubovsky, S.L. (1998) *Clinical psychiatry.* Washington, DC, American Psychiatric Association Press.

Duman, R.F., Heninger, C.R., and Nestler, E.J. (1997) A molecular and cellular theory of depression. Archives of General Psychiatry, 54, 597–606.

Feldman, R.S., Myer, J.S., and Quenzer, L.F. (1997) The Principles of Psychopharmacology. Sunderland, Massachusetts, Sinauer Associates Inc.

Gelenberg, A.J., and Bassuk, E.L. (1997) *The practitioners guide to psychoactive drugs, 4th edition.* New York, Plenum Medical Book Company.

Gorman, J.M. (1997) *Essential guide to psychiatric drugs 3rd edition.* St. Martin's paperback.

Guttmacher, L.B. (1994) *Psychopharmacology and electroconvulsive therapy.* Washington, DC, American Psychiatric Press, Inc.

Hardman, J.G., and Limbird, L.E. (1996) *Goodman and Gilman's the pharmacological basis of therapeutics,* 9th edition, New York, McGraw Hill.

Hyman, S.E. (1999) Introduction to the complex genetics of mental disorders. *Biological Psychiatry.* 45, 518–21.

Hyman, S.E., Arana, J.W., and Rosenbaum, J.F. (1995) *Handbook of psychiatric drug therapy, 3rd edition.* Boston, Little, Brown and Company.

International classification of diseases, 10th edition 0(ICD-10) classification of mental and behavioral disorders: clinical descriptions and diagnostic guidelines. World Health Organization, Geneva, 1993.

Janicak, P.G. (1999). *Handbook of psychopharmacology.* Philadelphia, Lippincott Williams & Wilkins.

Janicak, P.G., Davis, J.M., Preskorn, S.H., and Ayd, F.J. (1997) *Principles and practice of psychotherapy,* 2nd edition. Baltimore, Williams & Wilkins.

Jenkins, S.C., and Hansen, M.R. (1995) *A pocket reference for psychiatrists,* 2nd edition. Washington, DC, American Psychiatric Press, Inc.

Jensvold, M.F., Halbreich, U., and Hamilton, J.A. (1996) *Psychopharmacology and women.* Washington, DC, American Psychiatric Association Press.

Joffe, R.T., and Calabrese, J.R. (1994) *Anticonvulsants and mood disorders.* New York, Marcel Dekker, Inc.

Kaplan, H.I., Freedman, A.M., and Sadock, B.J. (1995) *Comprehensive textbook of psychiatry, 6th edition.* Baltimore, Williams & Wilkins.

Kaplan, H.I., and Sadock, B.J. (1993) *Pocket handbook of psychiatric drug treatment.* Baltimore, Williams & Wilkins.

Kaplan, H.I., Sadock, B.J., and Grebb, J.A. (1994) *Synopsis of psychiatry.* Baltimore, Williams & Wilkins.

Kramer, M.S., Cutler, N., Feighner, J. et al. (1998) *Distinct mechanism for antidepressant activity by blockade of central substance preceptors.* Science, 281, 640–5.

Journal of the American Academy of Child and Adolescent Psychiatry, Vol. 38(5), May 1995: *Special section: current knowledge in unmet needs in pediatric psychopharmacology.*

Kuitkin, F.M., Adams, D.C., Bowden, C.L., Heyer, E.J., Rifkin, A. et al. (1998) *Current psychotherapeutic drugs,* 2nd edition. Washington, DC, American Psychiatric Press, Inc.

Leonard, B.E. (1997) *Fundamentals of psychopharmacology.* Chichester, John Wiley & Sons.

Martindale, W. (1993) *The extra pharmacopoeia,* 30th edition, London, The Pharmaceutical Press.

Nelson, J.C. (Ed.) (1998) *Geriatric psychopharmacology.* New York, Marcel Dekker, Inc.

Nemoroff, C.B., and Schatzberg, A.F. (1999) *Recognition and treatment of psychiatric disorders: A psychopharmacology handbook for primary care.* Washington, DC, American Psychiatric Press.

Physician's desk reference, 49th edition. (1995) Montvale, NJ, Medical Economics Data Production Company.

Pies, R.W. (1998) *Handbook of essential psychopharmacology.* Washington, DC, American Psychiatric Press, Inc.

Practice guidelines for major depressive disorder in adults; American Psychiatric Association, Washington, DC, 1993.

Preskorn, S.H. (1999) *Outpatient management of depression,* 2nd edition. Caddo OK, Professional Communications Inc.

Prien, R.F., and Robinson, D.S. (Eds.) (1994) *Clinical evaluation of psychotropic drugs: principles and guidelines.* New York, Raven Press.

Robins, L.N., and Regier, D.A. (1991) *Psychiatric disorders in America: the epidemiologic catchment area study.* New York, The Free Press (Macmillan Inc.).

Schatzburg, A.F., and Cole, J.O. (1991) *Manual of clinical psychopharmacology*, 2nd edition, Washington, DC, American Psychiatric Press.

Schatzburg, A.F., Cole, J.O., and Debattista, C. (1997) *Manual of clinical psychopharmacology*, 3rd edition. Washington, DC, American Psychiatric Press, Inc.

Schatzburg, A.F., and Nemeroff, C.F. (Eds.) (1998) *Textbook of psychopharmacology*, 2nd edition, Washington, DC, American Psychiatric Press, Inc.

Shader, R.I. (1994) *Manual of psychiatric therapeutics.* Boston, Little, Brown and Company.

Stahl, S.M. (1997) *Psychopharmacology of antidepressants*, London, Dunitz Press.

Stahl, S.M. (1998) Basic psychopharmacology of antidepressants (part 1): antidepressants have seven distinct mechanisms of action. *Journal of Clinical Psychiatry* 59:(suppl 4) 5–14.

Stahl, S.M. (1998) Basic psychopharmacology of antidepressants (part 2): estrogen as an adjunct to antidepressant treatment. *Journal of Clinical Psychiatry* 59:(suppl 4) 15–24.

Stahl, S.M. (1998) Mechanism of action of serotonin selective reuptake inhibitors: serotonin receptors and pathways mediate therapeutic effects and side effects. *Journal of Affective Disorders* 12:215–235.

Stahl, S.M. (1999) *Psychopharmacology of antipsychotics*, London, Dunitz Press.

Taylor, D., McConnell, H., McConnell, D., Abel, K., and Kerwin, R. (1999) *The Bethlem and Maudsley NSH trust. Prescribing guidelines*, 5th edition. London, Martin Dunitz.

Walsh, B.P. (1998) *Child psychopharmacology.* Washington, DC, American Psychiatric Press, Inc.

INDEX

Note: Page numbers followed by f indicate illustrations; page numbers followed by t indicate tables.

Essential Psychopharmacology
Continuing Medical Education (CME)
Post Test
University of California
San Diego
Department of Psychiatry
School of Medicine

The University of California, San Diego School of Medicine is accredited by the Accreditation Council for Continuing Medical Education (ACCME) to sponsor continuing medical education (CME) programs for physicians. The University of California San Diego School of Medicine designates this continuing medical education activity for 14 hours of category I of the Physicians' Recognition Award of the American Psychiatric Association. Each physician should claim only those hours of credit he/she actually spent on the educational activity.

Instructions

This CME activity incorporates instructional design to enhance your retention of the didactic information and pharmacological concepts which are being presented. You are advised to go through this program unit by unit, in order, from beginning to end. You will first study the figures and read the figure legends for a single unit of instructional materials, and then go back and read the text that corresponds to that unit, reviewing the figures again as you go. After completing the text, you will then go back over the figures alone for another time. This will allow interaction with the materials, and also provide repeated exposure to the data and concepts presented both visually and in written explanations. Hopefully, this will be fun and interesting, and you will retain new information far more efficiently than you would after just reading the text or listening to a lecture on this topic.

Follow these directions to optimize your learning and retention of "Essential Psychopharmacology":

1. Go through each chapter unit one by one, from beginning to end and in order.
2. View each figure and read each figure legend.
3. Next, read the text while reviewing each figure as you go.

4. Complete the written post-test.
5. Review the figures once again checking any answers of which you are uncertain.
6. Photocopy and fill out the evaluation for the unit you just completed.
7. Fill out the CME registration form.
8. Pay $10 for each category I CME credit you are claiming (up to $140 for 14 credit hours).
9. Send the test answers, evaluations and check for the appropriate amount, payable to "UCSD Department of Psychiatry" to:

> Stephen M. Stahl, M.D., PH.D.
> Department of Psychiatry
> University of California San Diego
> 9500 Gilman Drive
> La Jolla, CA 92093-0603

REGISTRATION FORM FOR CME CREDIT

Essential Psychopharmacology (2nd Edition)
Stephen M. Stahl

Name of Registrant: _____

Address where CME certificate is to be sent:

_____

_____

_____

Number of category I CME credit hours claimed: _____
(CME fee: $10 for each credit hour; $295 discounted fee for all 54 credits)

Mail:
1. A check for the appropriate amount made payable to "UCSD, Department of Psychiatry" together with your answers and your evaluations

To:
> Stephen M. Stahl, M.D., Ph.D.
> Department of Psychiatry
> University of California, San Diego
> 9500 Gilman Drive
> La Jolla, CA 92093-0603

UNIT 5: DEPRESSION AND BIPOLAR DISORDERS*

Up to 6 Hours of Category 1 CME Credit

Objectives

1. To review the diagnostic criteria for depression and bipolar disorders.

2. To review the definitions of response, remission and recovery.

3. To learn the epidemiology and natural history as well as longitudinal course of depression.

4. To understand the biological basis of depression, including the monoamine hypothesis, the neurotransmitter receptor hypothesis and the hypothesis of reduced activation of brain neurotrophic factors.

5. To understand the functioning of noradrenergic, dopaminergic and serotonergic neurons.

Self Assessment and Post Test

1. The standard(s) usually targeted by studies seeking approval of most new antidepressants is (are):
   a. Response rates
   b. Remission rates
   c. Recovery rates
   d. Both a and b
   e. All of the above

2. Risk of relapse from depression is related to:
   a. The number of previous episodes
   b. Incomplete recovery
   c. Severity of index episode of depression
   d. Duration of index episode of depression
   e. All of the above

3. What is the best estimate for the risk of relapse into another episode of depression if an antidepressant is stopped within the first 6 to 12 months following a treatment response:
   a. Less than 5%
   b. At least 10%
   c. At least 33%
   d. At least 50%

*Please note that the numbers of the CME units given in this book refer to the chapter numbers they relate to in the full volume of *Essential Psychopharmacology*, second edition. Hence, in this volume, Chapter 1 relates to Unit 5, Chapter 2 relates to Unit 6, and Chapter 3 relates to Unit 7.

4. What is the best estimate for the risk of relapse into another episode of depression while taking an antidepressant for the first six months following a treatment response:
   a. Less than 5%
   b. At least 10%
   c. At least 33%
   d. At least 50%

5. The chances of a depressed patient responding to any known antidepressant is one out of three.
   a. True
   b. False

6. The chances of a depressed patient responding to a placebo is one out of three.
   a. True
   b. False

7. Presynaptic alpha 2 receptors:
   a. Control norepinephrine release
   b. Control serotonin release
   c. Both
   d. Neither

8. Which serotonin receptor(s) is (are) most involved with regulating the release of serotonin?
   a. 5HT1A
   b. 5HT1D
   c. 5TH2A
   d. Both a and b
   e. All the above

9. The locus coerulus is the principal location of the cell bodies of serotonergic neurons.
   a. True
   b. False

10. The locus coeruleus in the brainstem is the principal location of the cell bodies of nonadrenergic neurons.
    a. True
    b. False

11. The monoamine hypothesis of depression suggests that depression is predominantly caused by deficiency of serotonin.
    a. True
    b. False

12. The monoamine receptor hypothesis of depression suggests that depression is caused predominantly by an absence of key monoamine receptors in the brain.
    a. True
    b. False

13. The monoamine receptor hypothesis of gene activation suggests that depression is caused by:
    a. A problem in monoamines activating critical neuronal genes
    b. An inherited genetic deficiency in a specific gene for monoamines
    c. Stress-induced reduction in the expression of genes for neurotrophic factors such as BDNF
    d. a and c
    e. All of the above

14. The neurokinin neurotransmitters include:
    a. Substance P
    b. Neurokinins A and B
    c. Tachykinins 1 and 2
    d. a and b

15. Neurokinin receptor antagonists:
    a. Are effective in reducing pain
    b. Are potential antidepressants
    c. Are effective in reducing neurogenic inflammation

Evaluation

	Strongly Agree	Somewhat in Agreement	Neutral	Somewhat Disagree	Strongly Disagree
1. Overall the unit met my expectations.					
2. My general knowledge of depression was enhanced.					
3. The time spent reviewing the natural history and longitudinal course of depression was just right.					
4. The time spent reviewing neurotransmitter pharmacology was just right.					
5. The time spent reviewing biological theories of depression was just right.					
6. What topics would you like to see deleted or condensed from this unit?					

7. What topics would you like to see added or expanded in this unit?	
8. What is your overall opinion of this unit?	
9. What is your overall opinion of the usefulness of this unit to your clinical practice?	

UNIT 6: CLASSICAL ANTIDEPRESSANTS, SEROTONIN SELECTIVE REUPTAKE INHIBITORS AND NOREPINEPHRINE REUPTAKE INHIBITORS

Up to 4 Hours of Category I CME Credit

Objectives

1. To review the monoamine receptor hypothesis of depression.

2. To review the two classical categories of antidepressants, namely MAO inhibitors and tricyclic antidepressants.

3. To review the mechanism of action of the five serotonin selective reuptake inhibitors.

4. To review adrenergic modulators such as dopamine and norepinephrine uptake inhibitors.

5. To review selective inhibitors of norepinephrine reuptake.

6. To understand how drug actions can explain not only therapeutic effects but also side effects for antidepressants.

7. To review pharmacokinetic interactions of antidepressants with other drugs.

Self Assessment and Post Test

1. All antidepressants act by inhibiting the reuptake pump for serotonin, norepinephrine, or both.
   a. True
   b. False

2. When tricyclic antidepressants are given concomitantly with SSRIs such as fluoxetine or paroxetine:
   a. Plasma levels of the tricyclic antidepressants may rise
   b. Plasma levels of the tricyclic antidepressants may fall
   c. Plasma levels of fluoxetine or paroxetine may rise
   d. a and c

3. MAO inhibitors should not be administered concomitantly with:
   a. SSRIs (serotonin selective reuptake inhibitors)
   b. Meperidine
   c. Tyramine-containing foods
   d. All of the above

4. The mechanism of therapeutic action of SSRIs is:
   a. Stimulation of the serotonin transport pump
   b. Increasing the sensitivity of 5HT2A receptors
   c. Desensitizing somatodendritic 5HT1A autoreceptors
   d. None of the above

5. Side effects of the SSRIs such as anxiety, insomnia and sexual dysfunction may be mediated by stimulation of which serotonin receptor subtype?
   a. 5HT1A
   b. 5HT1D
   c. 5HT2A
   d. 5HT3

6. At high doses, which secondary property may apply to sertraline:
   a. 5HT2C agonist actions
   b. Blockade of dopamine transporters
   c. Blockade of muscarinic cholinegic receptors
   d. Blockade of cytochrome P450 1A2
   e. None of the above

7. At high doses, which secondary property may apply to fluoxetine:
   a. 5HT2C agonist actions
   b. Blockade of dopamine transporters
   c. Blockade of muscarinic cholinergic receptors
   d. Blockade of cytochrome P450 1A2
   e. None of the above

8. At high doses, which secondary property may apply to paroxetine:
   a. 5HT2C agonist actions
   b. Blockade of dopamine transporters
   c. Blockade of muscarinic cholinergic receptors
   d. Blockade of cytochrome P450 1A2
   e. None of the above

9. At high doses, which secondary property may apply to citalopram:
   a. 5HT2C agonist actions
   b. Blockade of dopamine transporters
   c. Blockade of muscarinic cholinergic receptors
   d. Blockade of cytochrome P450 1A2
   e. None of the above

10. The therapeutic action of bupropion is mediated in part via direct interactions with serotonergic neurotransmission.
    a. True
    b. False

11. The therapeutic action of reboxetine is mediated in part via direct interactions with serotonergic neurotransmission.
   a. True
   b. False

12. Increasing norepinephrine may cause:
   a. Antidepressant effects
   b. Improvement in attention
   c. Increase in motivation/reduction of apathy
   d. All of the above

Evaluation

	Strongly Agree	Somewhat in Agreement	Neutral	Somewhat Disagree	Strongly Disagree
1. Overall the unit met my expectations.					
2. My general knowledge about tricyclic antidepressants was enhanced.					
3. The time spent reviewing the pharmacology of classical antidepressants, including tricyclic antidepressants and MAO inhibitors, was just right.					
4. My general knowledge about serotonin selective reuptake inhibitors was enhanced.					
5. The time spent reviewing serotonin selective reuptake inhibitors was just right.					
6. What topics would you like to see added or expanded in this unit?					
7. What is your overall opinion of this unit?					
8. What is your overall opinion of the usefulness of this unit to your practice?					

Unit 7: Newer Antidepressants and Mood Stabilizers

Up to 4 Hours of Category I CME Credit

Objectives

1. To review the mechanism of action of dual reuptake inhibitors such as venlafaxine as well as other dual action antidepressants such as mirtazapine, and serotonin 2A antagonists such as nefazodone.

2. To review the mechanism of action of lithium and five anticonvulsants used as mood stabilizers (valproic acid, carbamazepine, lamotrigine, gabapentin and topiramate).

3. To discuss the use of antidepressants in combination with other drugs and antidepressants for the treatment of patients nonresponsive to monotherapies for depression and bipolar disorders.

Self Assessment and Post Test

1. Which of the following are serotonin 2A antagonists:
   a. Fluoxetine
   b. Nefazodone
   c. Paroxetine
   d. Mirtazapine
   e. b and d

2. Blocking a monoamine reuptake pump with an antidepressant can oppose the actions of drugs which block presynaptic alpha 2 receptors.
   a. True
   b. False

3. Dual neurotransmitter action at both serotonin and norepinephrine is possible only by combining two different psychopharmacological agents simultaneously.
   a. True
   b. False

4. Which of the following does not have selectivity for the noradrenaline transporter over the serotonin transporter:
   a. Desipramine
   b. Maprotiline
   c. Reboxetine
   d. Venlafaxine

5. Venlafaxine is a dual reuptake inhibitor of both serotonin and norepinephrine with equal potency for both transporters.
   a. True
   b. False

6. Lithium:
   a. Inhibits inositol monophosphatase
   b. Interacts with second messenger systems
   c. Blocks monoamine reuptake
   d. a and b
   e. All of the above

7. Which mood stabilizers are thought to act in part by interacting with ion channels:
   a. Carbamazepine
   b. Valproic acid
   c. Lithium
   d. a and b
   e. All of the above

8. Antidepressants can worsen depression in patients with bipolar disorders by inducing mania or rapid cycling.
   a. True
   b. False

9. Successful combinations of drugs for treating depressed patients resistant to monotherapies exploit pharmacologic synergies, where the total therapeutic effect may be greater than the sum of the parts.
   a. True
   b. False

10. The most accurate statement about psychotherapy for depression is that psychotherapy:
    a. Can be used instead of antidepressants for patients with marked to severe depression
    b. Has been proven to be useful for depression in all its different types, including psychodynamic, group cognitive, behavioral and psychoanalytical psychotherapies
    c. Has been demonstrated to be synergistic with antidepressants for standardized cognitive behavioral psychotherapy
    d. All of the above

Evaluation

	Strongly Agree	Somewhat in Agreement	Neutral	Somewhat Disagree	Strongly Disagree
1. Overall the unit met my expectations.					
2. My general knowledge about dual action antidepressants was enhanced.					

	Strongly Agree	Somewhat in Agreement	Neutral	Somewhat Disagree	Strongly Disagree
3. The time spent reviewing the pharmacology of venlafaxine, mirtazapine and nefazodone was just right.					
4. The time spent reviewing mood stabilizers was just right.					
5. The time spent reviewing antidepressant combinations was just right.					
6. What topics would you like to see deleted or condensed from this unit?					
7. What topics would you like to see added or expanded in this unit?					
8. What is your overall opinion of this unit?					
9. What is your overall opinion of the usefulness of this unit to your practice?					